THE HISTORY OF OTOSCLEROSIS TREATMENT

C'est une opération d'avenir. Il faudra, comme l'opération de la cataracte, attendre cent ans pour en apprécier la valeur.
E. Boucheron, La mobilization de l'étrier et son procédé opératoire, 1888

Sooner or later it is to be hoped the increase of the knowledge of the pathology of the conditions under discussion (otosclerosis) will bring about a revolution in the treatment of this disease.
A.A. Gray, Journal of Laryngology, Rhinology and Otology, 1906

Those who cannot remember the past are condemned to repeat it.
G. Santayana, The Life of Reason, 1905

THE HISTORY OF OTOSCLEROSIS TREATMENT

A survey of more than a century's search for the best treatment of the disease

R.A. Tange

ISBN: 978-90-6299-236-2

Distributors:
For the USA and Canada:
Pathway Book Service
4 White Brook Road
Gilsum, NH 03448, USA
pbs@pathwaybook.com

For all other countries:
Kugler Publications
P.O. Box 20538
1001 NM Amsterdam, The Netherlands
www.kuglerpublications.com

Kugler Publications is an imprint of SPB Academic Publishing bv, P.O. Box 20538, 1001 NM Amsterdam, The Netherlands

Table of Contents

Foreword

It is a great pleasure and honor to write this foreword. Prof. Tange has done an incredible amount of research into the theories of otosclerosis and the multitudes of treatments. He begins quoting G. Satayana: 'Those who cannot remember the past are condemned to repeat it.' This book is a must read for all of us who are treating patients with otosclerosis and for those who love the history of medicine.

The history of otosclerosis has a special place for me, as my father Howard P. House, MD was an early pioneer of otosclerosis surgery. During his training he was told not to diagnose otosclerosis as he was condemning the patient to progressive deafness. After finishing his residency in 1938 he traveled around the United States and Europe visiting various centers to learn from the giants in the field of Otolaryngology. While in Boston, Harris P. Moser, MD (Professor and Chairman at the Massachusetts Eye and Ear Infirmary) suggested that before departing for Europe he visit Julius Lempert, MD in New York. This visit changed his life. For the first time he saw a treatment that restored hearing: the one-stage endaural fenestration operation. Upon returning to Los Angeles in 1939 he was one of only two surgeons west of the Mississippi River performing the fenestration operation. Because of his visit with Lempert and the time he spent in Europe with other giants in the field, his practice became very busy. By 1947, he limited his practice to otology. His surgery schedule was booked for 18 months.

This book gives the history of otosclerosis from the 16th century to the present. Everyone will enjoy the reading and learning this fascinating history. In the late 1800's, our predecessors attempted to help their patients with innovative techniques and in some cases with disastrous results that included meningitis and death. These procedures included attempts to mobilize the stapes by placing a vibrator on the umbo of the malleus, blindly mobilizing the stapes through the tympanic membrane and even lateral semi-circular canal fenestration. All of these attempts were without magnification, poor illumination and antibiotics. Therefore, all further surgery for otosclerosis was condemned and no longer performed until the 1930's with early pioneers of the modern era.

Prof. Tange also includes a comprehensive section on a multitude of medical treatments for otosclerosis. I was amazed to learn that there were descriptions of trans-tympanic injections of thyroxin into the middle ear to prevent the advance or reverse the affects of otosclerosis. It is interesting to note that the results of so many of theses studies were more or less subjective as there were no audiometers. Therefore, the results were reported with the whisper test or the patient's subjective impressions. Also included as a comprehensive history of various listening devices including ear trumpets and bone conduction devices to improve communication for those suffering hearing loss due to otosclerosis.

As an avid fan of history I feel we can all improve our skills by gaining knowledge and inspiration of those who came before us. We have the advantage of learning from their ideas, successes and failures.

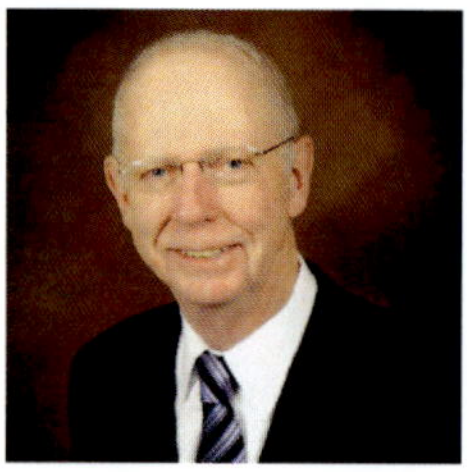

John W. House, MD

Preface

Hearing loss due to otosclerosis has been a subject of many different treatments. Since the understanding at the end of the nineteenth century that the disease was located in and around the cochlea and that it produces conducting and also perceptive hearing loss, all kinds of medical as well as surgical treatments have been applied to cure the disease. Most of the treatments have fallen into oblivion after the successful introduction of the stapedectomy in the late fifties of the last century. This book tries to highlight almost all possible treatments for otosclerosis presented in literature over the last hundred years. With the knowledge of today, many of the otosclerosis treatments of the past now seem absurd, but in reality generations of otosclerotic patients have been treated according to these treatments. The history of these treatments for otosclerosis shows the struggle of many well-meaning physicians and surgical ear pioneers to overcome the tragedy of the progression of the often genetic hearing loss due to otosclerosis. For those who are involved in the treatment of otosclerosis today, this historical overview will deepen the background of this specific ear disease and its forgotten treatments.

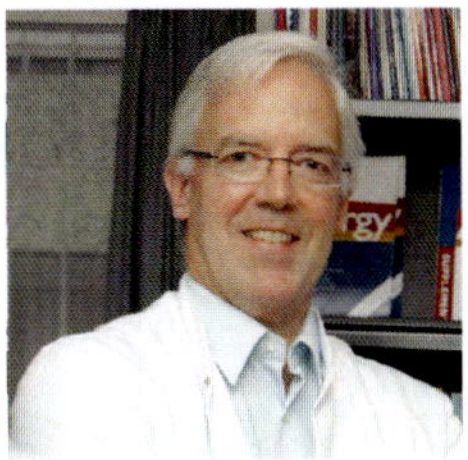

Rinze Anthony Tange

Chapter one

Introduction

1. Early history of stapes fixation and otosclerosis

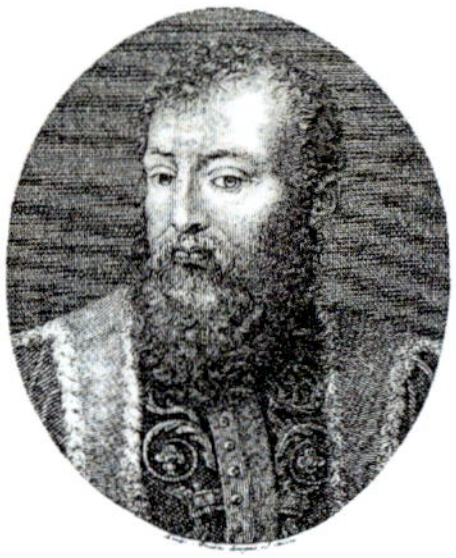

Fig. 1. Giovanni Filippo Ingrassia.

Otosclerosis is an affection of the middle and the inner ear. The stapes plays an important role in this affection. It was Giovanni Ingrassia (1510-1580; Fig. 1) who by accident discovered the stapes in the middle ear during cadaver studies.

The physiology of the hearing organ was described for the first time by Volcher Koyter (1534-1600). Hieronymus Capivacci († 1589) found a test to distinguish between perceptive and conducting hearing loss. It was Antonio Valsalva (1666-1723; Fig. 2a) who recognized the nature of the disease nowadays called otosclerosis. In his *De aure humana tractatus*, written while he was Professor of Anatomy at Bologna, he was the first to connect deafness during life with an ossified and fixed stapes found at autopsy (Fig. 2b).

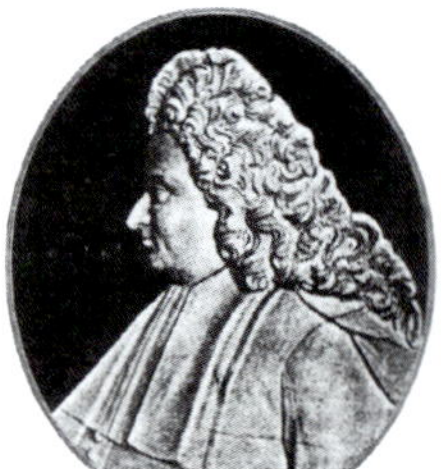

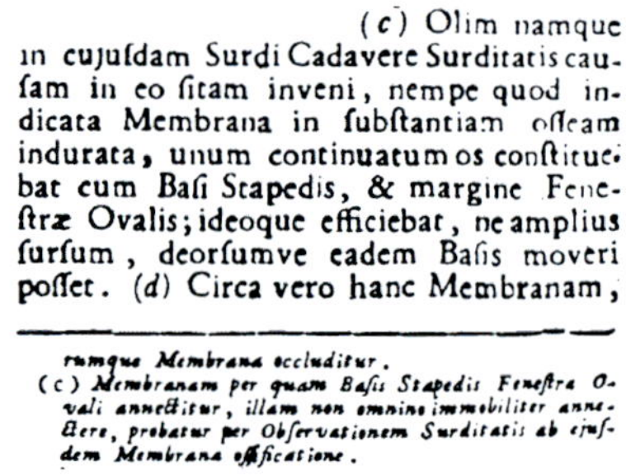

(c) Olim namque in cujusdam Surdi Cadavere Surditatis causam in eo sitam inveni, nempe quod indicata Membrana in substantiam osseam indurata, unum continuatum os constituebat cum Basi Stapedis, & margine Fenestræ Ovalis; ideoque efficiebat, ne amplius sursum, deorsumve eadem Basis moveri posset. (d) Circa vero hanc Membranam,

rumque Membrana occluditur.

(c) *Membranam per quam Basis Stapedis Fenestra Ovali annectitur, illam non omnino immobiliter annectere, probatur per Observationem Surditatis ab ejusdem Membrana officatione.*

Fig. 2a (left). Antonio Maria Valsalva.

Fig. 2b (right). Description of the stapes fixation by Valsalva (1724).

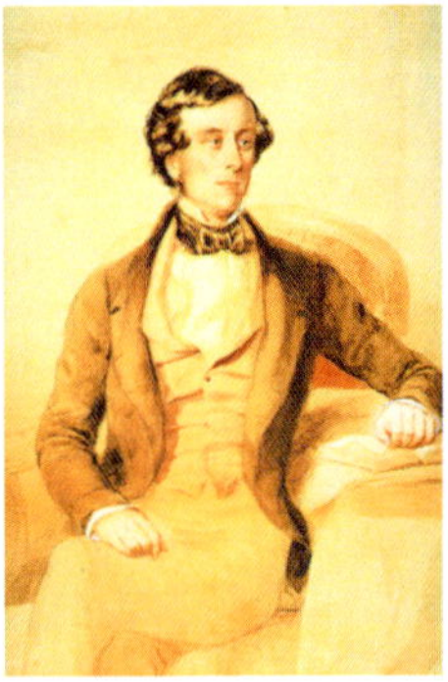

Fig. 3. Joseph Toynbee.

Valsalva gave the earliest description of the pathological otosclerotic process. Giovanni Morgagni (1761) refined the anatomical and pathological studies on the middle ear of his teacher Valsalva. Meckel (1771) and Domenico Cotugno demonstrated that there was fluid and no air inside the labyrinth. Joseph Toynbee of London (1815-1866; Fig. 3) focused attention upon the connection between stapes ankylosis and deafness after his study of 1659 human temporal bones in 1841. He found that in no less than 136 out of 1,149 dissected temporal bones, stapes ankylosis could be demonstrated. He distinguished four pathologic variations of stapes fixation. One of the first observations of an otosclerotic focus at the stapes footplate was by Adam Politzer in 1862 (Fig. 4). He described a case of white bony formation at the place of an immobile stapes footplate in a cadaver.

Politzer could not explain the etiology of the process leading to the new bone formation and fixation of the stapes in human temporal bones. Because of the lack of signs of infection around the stapes in his histological slides, he stated that the ankylosis of the stapes could not be regarded as a result of middle-ear infections.

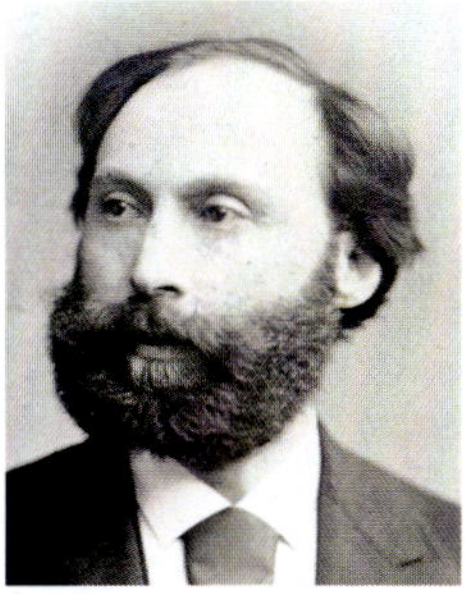

Figs. 4a & 4b. Adam Politzer (1835-1920; above) and his observance of the histology of otosclerosis (below).

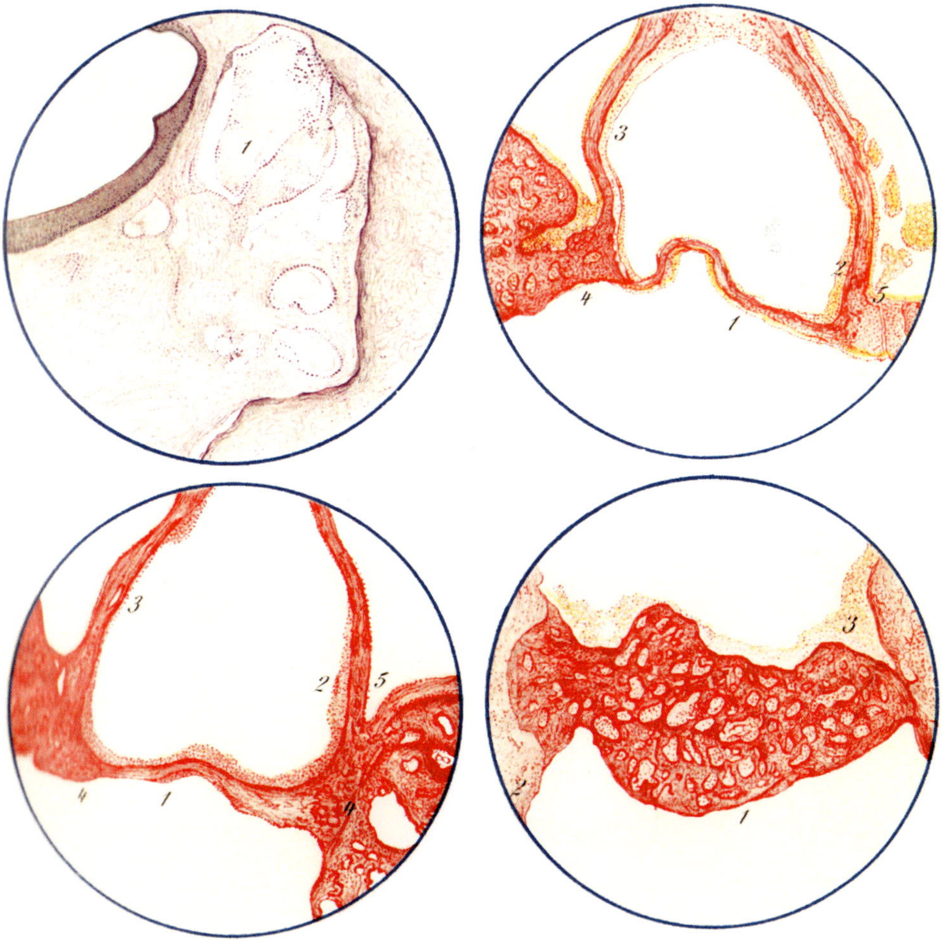

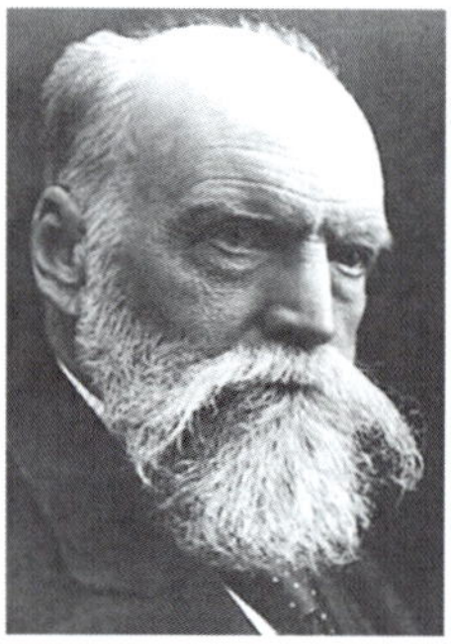

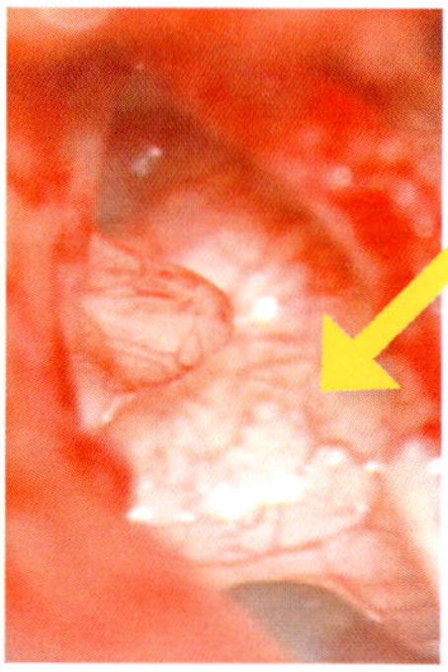

Figs. 5a & 5b. Hermann Hugo Rudolf Schwartze (left); Schwartze's sign, visible during middle ear exploration (right). Note the increased vascularity of the cochlear promontary (arrow).

Schwartze (1837-1910; Fig. 5) described in 1870 the reddish discoloration behind the tympanic membrane and later he found an increased vascularity of the cochlear promontary during the active stage of otosclerosis. This phenomenon later became known as 'Schwartze's sign', and it occurs in about 10% of otosclerosis ears. Von Troltsch (1881) used the term 'sclerosis' for stapes fixation. He thought that sclerosis of the tympanic cavity mucosa caused stapes fixation.

It was in 1890 that L. Katz from Ludwighaven gave a first full pathological report together with the results of the clinical examination of the patient with otosclerosis and finally filled in the completed clinical picture of the disease. He found microscopic evidence of otosclerosis resulting in stapes fixation. In 1893, Politzer described otosclerosis as a clinical entity and further characterized its pathology as a 'primary disease of the bony labyrinthine capsule', in which neoplastic bone gradually takes the place of normal bone, and produces ankylosis of the stapes.

2. Early conservative and surgical treatments of otosclerosis

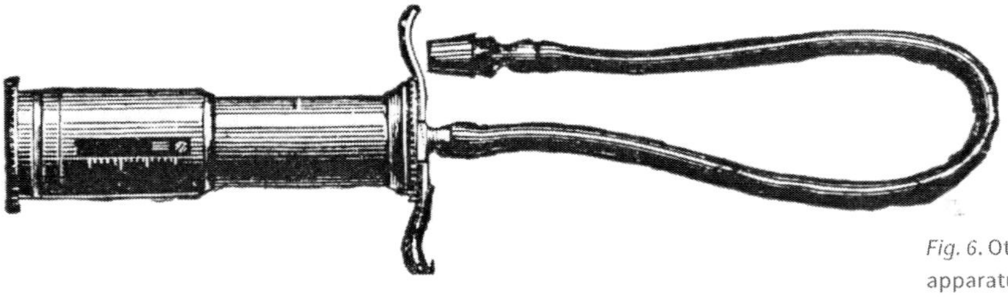

Fig. 6. Oto-massage apparatus by Delstanche.

The classic conservative treatment was focused on the remobilization of the ossicular hearing chain. Inflation using Politzer's balloon was invented with the object of causing forced movement of the ossicular chain so that the stapes would be rendered mobile in the oval window. Oto-massage of the eardrum with the ossicular chain was performed by Delstanche from Brussels, to exercise the ossicles and halt the process causing the immobilization. He designed an apparatus which changes the pressure on the eardrum by closing the external canal and then changing the pressure (Fig. 6). In 1899, at the sixth International

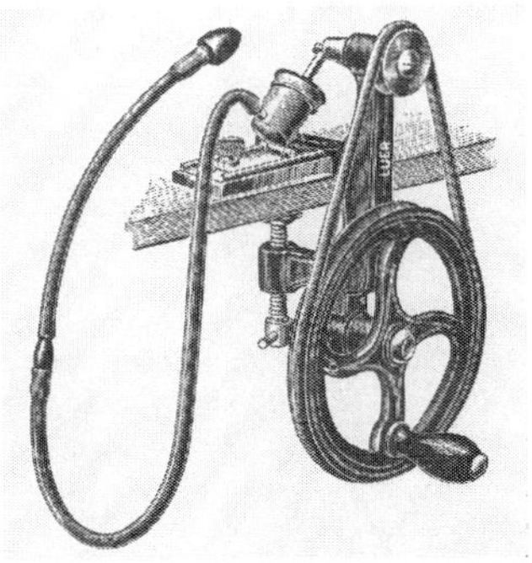

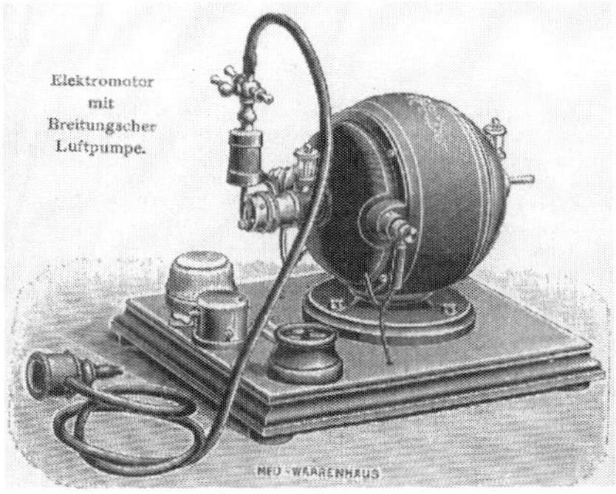

Figs. 7 & 8. Breitung's oto-massage apparatuses: hand-powered (left) and powered by electricity (right).

Otologic Congress in London, his invention was awarded with the Lenval prize. Breitung made an airpump with positive and negative pressure which came into force by a pinion and in a later version by electric power (Figs. 7 & 8). These oto-massage apparatuses formed the basis for the later development of the

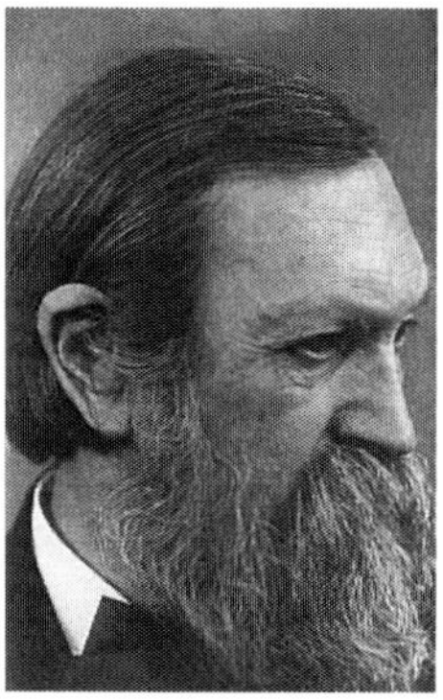

Fig. 9. Ernst Mach.

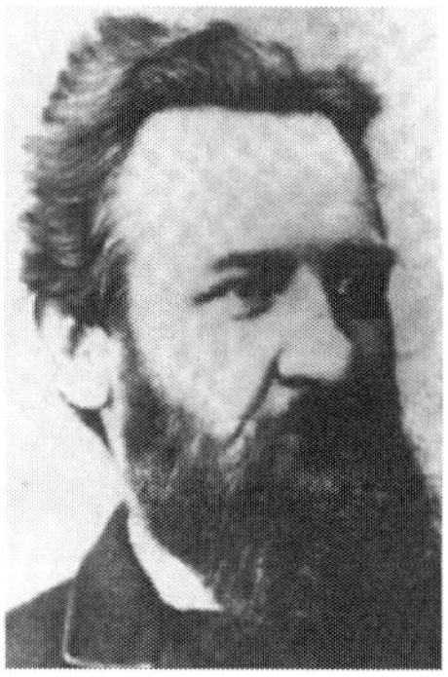

Fig. 10. Johannes Kessel.

re-education machines like the Kinesiphone and Zünd-Burguet electrophonoïd.

Injection of vaseline or pepsin solution in the middle ear, the use of vibrating probes and insufflations of the middle ear were other treatments to mobilize the ankylosis of the stapes. These treatments were successful for a short time, but often resulted in tuba obstruction and middle-ear infections. Because Toynbee believed that the whole disease was due to rheumatism or gout, he treated patients according to these conditions and stated to be successful in improving hearing. Bacon in 1898 recommended administration of large doses of iodide or potash, which should be kept up for a year or more to stop the ankylosis of the stapes. These conservative methods of treatment of the stapes ankylosis were not successful. With the early recognition that the process was in fact an immobilizing of the stapes in the oval window, many treatments were used experimentally without a full clinical appreciation of the actual process.

Because of the failure of these conservative methods, surgical intervention for the problem became an option. Ernst Mach (1838-1916; Fig. 9) from Prague was probably the first to perform a mobilization of the stapes in 1875.

After experimental operations on dog and pigeon, Kessel (1839-1907; Fig. 10) performed his stapes mobilization and extraction operation in 1876. The problem of the mobilization of the stapes was the approach straight through the tympanic membrane. Kessel decided to go directly to the stapes footplate after ablation of the membrane and the middle ear ossicles after an antroatticotomy. Because in many cases the results were not satisfactory, Kessel also extracted the stapes. Ear surgery at that time was not without danger. There were no microscopes or antibiotics available, which meant that there was a great risk of – often fatal – meningitis. Furthermore, a facial-nerve palsy and intensive bleeding could occur. J. Michel from Grenoble also published his experience with the mobilization, in 1876 (Willemot, 1981).

Lucae (1835-1911; Fig. 11a) from Berlin described a technique for the mobilization of the stapes by repeated percussion of the ossicular chain in 1884. He designed a very tiny pressure probe (see Fig. 11b) to place on the malleus handle at the umbo of the eardrum. With his method he was able to mobilize the hearing chain by hand. The method was not successful because the

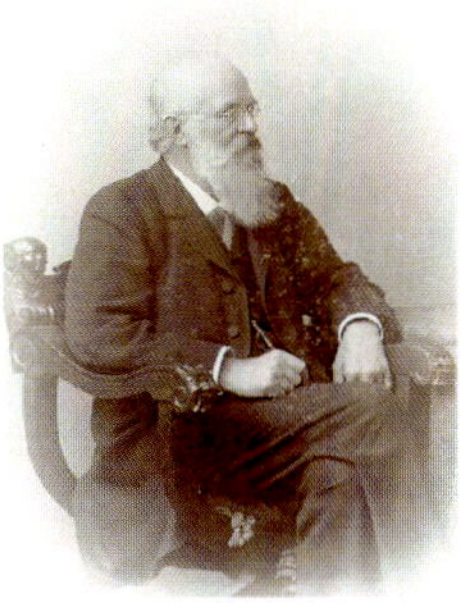

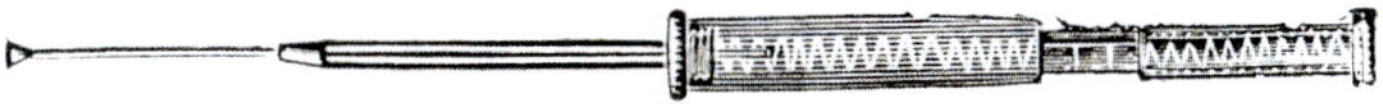

Figs. 11a & 11b. Johann Constantin August Lucae (above) and his pressure probe for chain mobilization. (left)

Table 1. The pioneers of otosclerosis surgery in the 19th century.

Surgeon	Year	Place	Result
Mach	1875	Prague	First mobilization of the stapes
Kessel	1876	Jena	Mobilization of the stapes
Michel	1876	Grenoble	Mobilization of the stapes
Lucae	1884	Berlin	Repeated percussion of the chain
Boucheron	1888	Paris	60 cases, good results/frequent infections
Gellée	1888	Paris	Blind mobilization through membrane
Sexton	1889	New York	Removal of the stapes
Schwartze	1890	Halle	42% success
Blake	1890	Boston	Good results but not long-lasting
Jack	1892	Boston	Good results but not long-lasting
Miot	1896	Paris	24/18 = 75% success
Anderston	1896	New York	Footplate perforation with dental drill
Floderus	1899	Denmark	Fistula in semicircular canal
Faraci	1899	Palermo	Success in a few cases
Ballance	1900	London	Fistula in semicircular canal

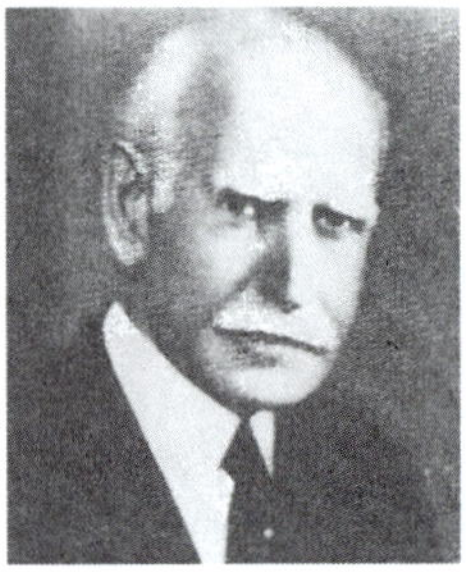
Fig. 12. Frederick L. Jack.

treatment was too painful and the hearing did not improve. E. Boucheron from Paris published 60 cases of stapes mobilization with a success lasting more then sixteen months in 1888. Unfortunely, there were frequent infections in most of the cases. Boucheron was some kind of prophet when he wrote about the stapes mobilization: *'C'est une opération d'avenir. Il faudra, comme l'opération de la cataracte, attendre cent ans pour en apprécier la valeur.'* Miot from Paris reported in 1896 on 126 cases of mobilization of the stapes, 24 cases of which were otosclerosis. In 18 of the 24 cases a good result was demonstrated. In the USA, C.J. Blake and F.L. Jack (1861-1951; Fig. 12) from Boston and J.H. Burnett from Philadelphia reported remarkable improvement in hearing after removal of the stapes. The results were not long-lasting. In only a few cases the result remained stable after ten years after the surgery.

The surgical approach to the fixated stapes in otosclerosis was unsuccessful due to recurrent infections and the risk of intracranial abscesses. To avoid the actual focus of disease, K.A. Passow (1897) from Heidelberg made an opening to the cochlea in the medial wall of the middle ear close to the oval window. The promontory was trephined and the opening covered with a mucoperiosteal flap. No lasting improvement was obtained, and often the hearing was made worse. H.A. Alderston (1896) from New York tried to drill with a dental drill through the stapes footplate to create a fistula, but the results of this procedure were without lasting success.

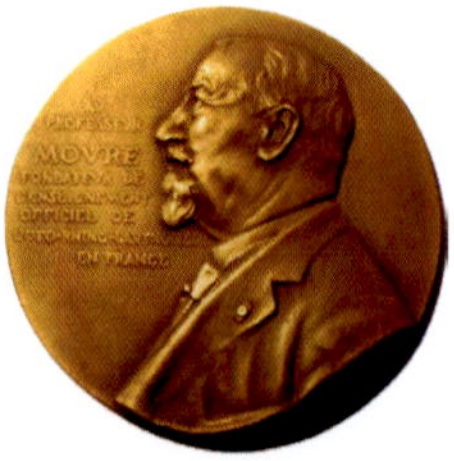
Fig. 13. Medal with the portrait of Emile Moure.

B. Floderus from Denmark in 1898 and C.A. Ballance in 1900 were the first suggesting the creating of a fistula into the horizontal semicircular canal to stop vertigo problems and in some cases to improve hearing. By accident, Ballance opened the horizontal semicircular canal during mastoid surgery. He covered the fistula by a thin layer of squamous epithelium skin transplant and observed that the pre-operative vertigo was diminished and the hearing improved. Recurrent infections were an important reason that these fistulae operations for otosclerosis were unsuccessful.

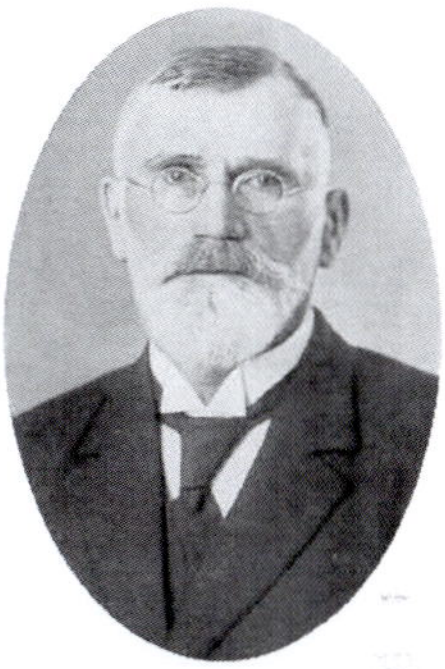

Fig. 14. Friedrich Siebenmann.

In 1894, on an international congress on medicine in Rome, V. Cozzolino, E. Moure (1855-1914; Fig. 13) and A. Politzer condemned the surgery on the stapes in cases of otosclerosis. F. Bacon reports in his *Manual of Otology* (1898) that operations on the stapes should not be considered for a moment. In 1900, two other leading authorities at that time, F. Siebenmann (1852-1928; Fig. 14) and R.D. Botey, condemned the surgical treatment of otosclerosis at the International Congress of Otology again in Rome. In that pre-antibiotics era, an operation for hearing loss with the possible side effect of often fatal meningitis was the reason not to perform the surgery for hearing improvement in otosclerosis. Politzer stated, also in 1900, that the simple mobilization of the stapes only results in a temporary effect on the hearing and that operative extraction of the stapes was of no use

Table 2.

Year	Those who condemned stapes surgery	Where
1894	Cozzolino, Moure and Politzer	Congress – Rome
1898	Bacon	Manual of Otology
1900	Siebenmann, Botey	Congress – Rome
1900	Politzer	Publication
1904	Denker	His book – *Otosklerose*

and could even be dangerous. In 1904, A. Denker (1863-1941) from Munich declared that there was no future for the surgical treatment of deafness due to otosclerosis. Since these statements (Table 2) at the beginning of the twentieth century and the poor results at that time, stapes surgery was abandoned for almost more than two decades as treatment for otosclerosis. Because of this fact, medical treatment of otosclerosis became an option.

Chapter two

Non-surgical treatment of otosclerosis

1. Medical treatment of otosclerosis

1.1. Treatment of the endocrine system for retardation of the otosclerosis process

In 1912, Voss suggested the possibility of a relationship between otosclerosis and disturbances of the function of the parathyroid gland. Since then, various investigations have been published with the object of demonstrating metabolic disturbances of different kinds in association with the disease otosclerosis. W. Sohier Bryant from New York (1915) believed that the cerebral pituitary, the suprarenals, the parathyroid glands, and the ovaries have an strong relation to otosclerosis. There have also been reports on investigations of the inorganic phosphate, cholesterol and protein contents of the serum, as well as a few publications on the serum potassium, magnesium, chlorine and lactic acid, the alkali reserve, the sugar metabolism and the basal metabolism in relation with otosclerosis. P. Manasse (1912) has found in cases of goitre bone changes similar to those in otosclerosis. Improvement in otosclerosis has been noted after the administration of thyroid extract. In those days, the attention was particularly focused on the calcium metabolism and the parathyroid function. A parathyroid insufficiency was assumed as an important factor in the causation of otosclerosis. H. Leicher (1928) in an exhaustive survey of the subject, suggested parathyroid transplantation for otosclerosis. H. Frey and A. Kriser (1923) reported good results for the treatment of otosclerosis from the applications of X-rays to the parathyroid glands. Very favorable results were reported by E. Watson-Williams (1929) in a case study of five patients who were treated for otosclerosis with commercial parathyroid tablets. It was claimed that the treatment was simple, safe, inexpensive and did not interfere with ordinary work. Otosclerosis has also been treated with ultra-violet light, and some very good results have been reported. L. Mirvish (1925) believed that otosclerosis was due to hypoparathyroidism, so he started to treat three otosclerotic patients with parathormone injections (Lilly) while their hearing was continuously controlled by quantitative hearing tests during one to three years. Although the group studied was very small, the results were promising: in one case the progress of deafness was arrested, while in the other cases a considerable improvement in hearing was achieved. A.A. Gray in 1935 believed that otosclerosis could be cured by local application of thyroxine in the middle ear. The method employed in the application of thyroxine to the ear consists of injecting the drug, suspended in four minims of distilled water, through the tympanic membrane into the middle ear by means of an ordinary well-made and smoothly working hypodermic syringe. Fourteen cases were treated and very considerable improvement was achieved in seven of these cases (50%). Of these seven patients, the tinnitus was greatly relieved in those who presented with that symptom. The subjective symptom of paracusis, usually considered of very unfavorable significance, was no contra-indication to this method of treatment, as two of the most successful cases were the ones with paracusis. All these attempts to treat otosclerosis, however, were inconclusive, because in most of the cases the period of observation was not long enough, and the reported improvement in hearing had been judged by the patients' own observations. Due to the hypothesis on the otosclerosis pathogenesis that a disregulation of the calcium metabolism by the parathyroid glands creates otosclerotic nests around the cochlea, a surgical solution by a parathyroidectomy was introduced. This parathyroid trouble was called dysparathyroidsm, and the treatment was the removal of the left parathyroid gland by ligature of the arteries to these gland, resulting in a decrease of gland secretion. According to this theory, removal of the left parathyroid gland should stop the otosclerotic process. Alonzo and Chiarino performed their first parathyroid surgery for the treatment of otosclerosis in Uruguay and presented their results in august 1936 in Berlin. They reported a total of 19 cases of otosclerosis in which parathyroidectomy resulted in an almost immediate improvement in hearing, which, however, decreased slowly. Long-term results of this treatment of otosclerosis are unknown.

The upcoming success of the fenestration surgery for otosclerosis in those days must have been the reason that the parathyroidectomy as treatment for otosclerosis was soon forgotten.

1.2. Sex hormones and treatment of otosclerosis

Conrad Stein (1925) made a careful study of 125 cases of otosclerosis, and came to the conclusion that there was definitely a connection between sexual functions and disturbances and the onset of otosclerosis. For example, 31/85 = 36% of the females with otosclerosis suffered from menstrual disorders. Of the ten male patients who started to suffer from otosclerosis at puberty, two suffered from hypoplasia, one from hyperplasia of the genital organs, and one from hypospadias. Other patients presented with histories of neurasthenia, accompanied by impotence, frigidity, and other derangements of a normal sexual life. So Stein concluded that in nearly every case otosclerosis was associated with conditions of nervous degeneration, particularly in connection with sexual abnormalities, and that therefore disturbances of the secretion of the endocrine glands must be responsible for the disease. This causation of otosclerosis was therefore believed to have a connection in some way with the sexual organs like the ovaries and testicles. This supposition was based on certain peculiarities of the disease, especially its preponderance in females. The disease often begins at puberty and the hearing loss could become worse during each pregnancy. So some otologists reasoned they could test administration of sex hormones as a treatment for otosclerosis. J. Bernstien (aural surgeon) and L. Gillis (1939) tried administration of sex hormones because these hormones cause dilatation of the peripheral vessels and an increased circulation of blood. This increased peripheral circulation might cause absorption of the embryonic bone present in otosclerosis lesions. Fifty-six otosclerosis cases (38 females and 18 males) were treated with sex hormones. The results of the study were published in *Lancet*. All patients were treated with injections of sex hormones, some consisting of homogenic hormones and others of heterogenic hormones. The authors documented the changes in hearing, in many cases without the patient's knowledge, to test the effects of the different hormones. The hearing of the patients was tested with the spoken voice, the whispered voice, and the tuning-fork. An audiometer was not available at the time of the investigation. Tests with the spoken voice and whispered voice provided sufficient information about any changes in hearing. Also the information and the opinions of the patients' friends and relations were considered of importance for the results of the treatment. An improvement of hearing was obtained in 31 of their 56 patients. Better results were obtained in females (24/38 = 63%) compared to the male patients (7/18 = 38%). In most cases, the heterogenic hormone was responsible for the improvement. Six illustrative cases (three males and three females) were presented. Different sex hormones like Progynon and Testoviron from Schering and Oestrone and Perandren from CIBA were injected weekly for seven to twelve weeks. Side effects of the treatment were not documented. The authors believed that the duration of their study was sufficient to show the efficacy of the treatment; since the usual course of otosclerosis was progressive deterioration of hearing, any improvement was considered a great advantage. The authors were convinced that their results were promising enough to encourage further investigation. M. Yearsley abstracted the publication and noticed that there was no literature search of previous work on the subject. In a commentary in *Lancet* on the publication of the sex hormones in otosclerosis by J. Bernstien and L. Gillis it was regretted that the audiometer was not used in this investigation, for the voice was not a sufficiently reliable method of testing hearing results. It was to be hoped by the editor that others will give the method a stricter trial. It was concluded that in the past diverse methods have been advocated for the treatment of the intractable condition of otosclerosis, accompanied by encouraging case-reports, but most of these methods did sunk again into oblivion afterwards. This fear also became truth for after this sole publication on sex hormones as treatment for otosclerosis no papers on this subject have been appeared in literature.

1.3. Cortisone treatment in otosclerosis

The use of cortisone in arthritis gave rise to hopes that good results could be obtained by this drug in the treatment of otosclerosis. Because of the theoretical similarity between the joint fixation in arthritis and the stapedial fixation in many cases of otosclerosis, cortisone and corticotropin were accordingly given in trials. However, the results were disappointing. Corticotropin (ACTH) has been applied intramuscularly in a small series of cases of otosclerosis studied by N. Riskaer (1951). The results of this study of unoperated otosclerosis cases showed no effect on hearing after several years of follow up. V. Goodhill (1952) tested the effect of oral cortisone on a series of fenestrated otosclerosis patients post-operatively after fenestration surgery. The cortisone therapy did not change the hearing. A temporary subjective improvement due to elation and euphoria was observed post-operatively. Local treatment of the fenestration cavity by cortisone has been applied by C.A. Hutchinson (1954), resulting in accelerated healing of the cavity and a shorter hospital stay. K.B. Sachdev and M.L. Bhatia (1962) suggested local treatment of the middle ear for otosclerosis by means of Eustachian tube catheterization. They treated 42 otosclerotic ears of 25 patients by insufflating the middle ear with three different corticosteroids: Decadron, Efcorlin and Hydroxylcortisone. They noted an overall improvement of hearing in 36% of cases. Decadron and Hydroxycortisone were found to be more effective than Efcorlin. Notwithstanding their enthusiasm for this new method of conservative therapy in clinical otosclerosis, this treatment for otosclerosis also disappeared. More recently H. Riechelmann *et al.* (2000) evaluated the efficiency of prophylactic peri-operative glucocorticoid treatment during stapes surgery in preventing damage to the inner ear and reducing the frequency of early post-operative complications. Ninety-five consecutive patients undergoing erbium:YAG laser-assisted stapedotomy for otosclerosis were included in their study. The result of this prospective, randomized, unblinded study was that peri-operative cortisone prophylaxis for prevention of inner ear damage during stapes surgery was ineffective and associated with increased postoperative patient discomfort. Cortisones were also used as treatment after unsuccessful stapes surgery with deafness (H.P. Beales, 1987). Together with repeated injections of nicotinic acid intravenously or intravenous heparin in small doses, hydrocortisone was used, in gradually decreasing doses, as it was believed that it protected the inner ear cell membranes, and had an anti-inflammatory, anti-edematous and anti-haemorrhagic effects. Sodium fluoride was sometimes added to this basic treatment for an anti-enzymatic effect on the cochlear lesions. In literature, positive results from this treatment of otosclerosis are lacking.

1.4. Fluoride therapy

S.R. Guild in 1944 showed that in one out of eight women and in one out of fifteen men otosclerosis occurred in their temporal bone and that in only 10% of those cases a conductive deafness due to stapedial fixation could be demonstrated. This pure cochlear otosclerosis with senso-neural hearing loss was difficult to treat. Studies have shown that in the active otosclerotic phase, resorption of mature lamellar bone by osteoclasts occurs with replacement by osteoblastic disposition of a collagenous matrix. This subsequent mineralization leads to the formation of immature bone of increased thickness, vascularity and cellularity. D.S. Bernstein and colleagues (1966) demonstrated that in areas where the population used water with a higher content of fluoride less osteoporosis occurred. H.J. Daniel (1969) demonstrated that stapes fixation due to otosclerosis occurred more often in areas with low fluoride in the drinking water compared with areas with a high content of fluoride. In Australia, R.E. Gristwood was able to establish that a high incidence (30%) of obliterated stapes footplates correlated with an extremely low fluoride concentration. Because of the similarity of osteoporosis and otosclerosis and the findings of the relation between the concentration of fluoride in drinking water and otosclerosis, G.E. Shambaugh Jr. and A. Scott (1964) suggest that sodium fluoride, given in moderate to high doses, might influence favorably the otosclerostic bone lesions. The concept of this type of treatment was that sodium fluoride might promote the change of actively expanding otosclerotic lesions to more dense, inactive lesions. The fluoride stimulated the natural tendency of otosclerotic lesions to become recalcified and inactive. The result of this treatment would be a stabilization of the progressive sensorineural deafness due to otosclerosis, a reduction of tinnitus and an improvement of mild vestibular symptoms. Several concepts have been published in the last 35 years about the mode of action of sodium fluoride. D.T. Cody and H.L. Baker, and later G.B. Brookes, recommended vitamin D and calcium as adjuvants to the fluoride therapy for otosclerosis. In a study of 45 patients treated that way, one case showed a spectacular improvement of bone conduction hearing to vitamin D and calcium in conjunction with fluoride. Reduction of osteoclastic bone resorption and stimulating of osteoblastic bone formation by sodium fluoride has been demonstrated in animal experimental studies. Bretlau *et al.* (1981) reported on an evaluation of sodium fluoride treatment using scanning transmission electron microscopy together with an energy dispersive x-ray element analyser. The results showed that using the calcium/phosphorus ratio as an indication for bone maturity, sodium fluoride could stabilize otosclerotic lesions, particularly the spongiotic type with unstable mineralization, in retaining calcium relative to phosphorus. Sodium fluoride seems to promote recalcification and to reduce the activity of otospongiotic bone. An anti-enzymatic action of sodium fluoride was introduced by Causse *et al.* (1980). When the balance between trypsin and α1-antitrypsin is disturbed in favor of trypsin, this results in an increase of trypsin values that damage the hair cells, leading to cochlear hearing loss. It was shown that sodium fluoride can act directly on trypsin and reduces the levels of protease inhibitors. It was accepted that the overall reduction of enzymatic rates by inhibition favors the stabilization of the otosclerotic process and consequential arrest or slowing down the cochlear deterioration. These findings were supported by other authors. In a clinical report on a large series of over 5000 patients treated with sodium fluoride, Causse *et al.* (1993) found that medical treatment with sodium fluoride results in a stabilization of cochlear deterioration in the majority of cases. Only a few patients showed an improvement in sensorineural hearing. Furthermore it was found that sodium fluoride seems to slow conductive hearing loss by stapedial fixation. In a prospective clinical double-blind, placebo-controlled study of 95 patients by Bretlau *et al.* it has been statistically shown that perceptive hearing loss was significantly worse in non-treated otosclerotic patients compared with patients treated with 40 mg fluoride daily. Another study on the effect of fluoride therapy by Colleti *et al.* demonstrated that sodium fluoride (NaF) had a stabilizing effect on early otosclerosis and that fluoride arrests the disease process in more than 60% of ears at the two-year follow up and in more than 50% at five years follow up. They suggested a program of secondary prevention of otosclerosis by fluoride. Freeman (1980) demonstrated that sodium fluoride therapy could be beneficial not only in controlling the progressive sensorineural hearing loss, but also the symptoms of vestibular dysfunction in patients with cochlear otosclerosis. Despite these positive findings and studies, the administration of sodium fluoride remains a matter of controversy, partly because of the known and unknown toxic effect of long-term medication with sodium fluoride. In 1989, Kerr regarded the use of fluoride in otosclerosis therapy as experimental, despite reports of the efficacy. On the other hand, Chamyal *et al.* (1990) believed that NaF should be administered pre-operatively in cases of otosclerosis with pulsatile nature of tinnitus and a positive Schwartze sign. If overall stabilization of the otosclerosis occurred then the patients are expected to maintain a life-long fluoride therapy. According to Shambaugh *et al.* (1980) and Causse *et al.* (1993), stopping treatment in those patients whose disease process stabilized during therapy, may result in a reactivation of the disease in two to three years. The long-term NaF therapy, however, is not without negative consequences. In 42% of the patients treated by 50 mg/day NaF for osteoporosis, Riggs *et al.* (1980) observed side effects of the treatment. This dose of 50 mg/day NaF is the same as in the treatment for severe cochlear otosclerosis. Arthralgia and painful plantar faciitis were the most common side effects noticed. Side effects of the oral treatment by sodium fluoride for otosclerosis have been documented as a high incidence of dyspeptic symptoms like nausea, vomiting, gastritis and peptic ulcer. Also bone pain and exostosis formation have been seen as side effect of NaF treatment. The treatment had to be stopped when gastric distress occurred (Uppal *et al.*, 2010). Contra-indications for the treatment are renal impairment and pregnancy. Because of the possible side effects, a regular follow up is necessary. For example, serum levels of calcium, phosphate and alkaline phosphate must be checked and skeleton imaging must be performed to detect fluorosis. Besides these precautions, regular hearing testing during therapy is important to check if the progression of hearing loss is stopped. All these precautions make this medical treatment rather laborious and for the patient burdensome. In the light of these precautions, the side effects and the fact that there are still doubts that oral NaF interrupts the cochlear otosclerotic process, one can wonder if there is still a place for this treatment of cochlear otosclerosis. Most studies showing favorable results are not randomized and only a few studies are carried out as double-blind randomized, placebo-controlled trials. In studies by Vartiainen *et al.* (1997) it was shown that long-term fluoridation of drinking water did not influence the bone conduction in cases of otosclerosis significantly. Browning (2008) stated that there is no evidence at present that the level of fluoride in drinking water has an impact on progression of clinical otosclerosis and that there is also no evidence that the use of oral sodium fluoride interrupts the cochlear otosclerotic process. Recently, Cruise *et al.* (2010) published a literature review on the subject of fluoride therapy for cochlear otosclerosis, and their conclusion was that there was not enough evidence suggesting that sodium fluoride may be of benefit to preserve hearing and to reduce vestibular symptoms in patients with otosclerosis. Sodium-fluoride therapy has been shown to have some beneficial effect on dizziness associated with otosclerosis. In view of the possibility of systemic side effects of sodium-fluoride therapy, a regular follow up of patients is required. Bisphosphonates can be considered as an alternative treatment to sodium fluoride in cases where the patient is intolerant to sodium-fluoride therapy.

1.5. Bisphosphonate treatment

Causse *et al.* (1982) suggested that bisphosphonates could function as an alternative treatment for the use of sodium fluoride in cochlear otosclerosis. Bisphosphonates are medicines that target the reduction of osteoclasts by accelerating their cell death. Bisphosphonates could be considered as a new follow-up product to sodium fluoride for medical treatment of otosclerosis. They were introduced in 1985 by Stutzmann and Petrovic. Kennedy (1993) performed a two-year prospective double-blind study to evaluate the role of the bisphosphonate etidronate disodium for the treatment of progressive hearing loss in patients with otosclerosis. A pulsed dosage regimen was used during a two-year period and the patients were followed up with otologic and audiometric examinations. No statistically significant differences were achieved between the study and control groups. The study showed, however, a trend towards stabilization or improvement in air conduction thresholds in some frequencies (1000 and 4000 Hz) and in bone conduction thresholds at other frequencies (500, 1000, and 2000 Hz). The incidence of adverse side effects was similar in the treatment and control groups. Brookler and Tanyeri (1997) presented their experience with bisphosphonate treatment for otosclerosis in a retrospective case-review study. The efficacy of etidronate was assessed as a treatment for the inner ear symptoms of otosclerosis in a retrospective case review of 896 patients diagnosed with otosclerosis, with primary complaints of dizziness, hearing loss, tinnitus or Meniere's syndrome. The diagnosis of otosclerosis was based on small-pixel computed tomography of the temporal bones. Of the 896 patients placed on an etidronate protocol, 545 were followed for more than six months and were analyzed. The symptomatic response to etidronate, as well as audiologic and computerized rotary chair results were used in the assessment. Patients who were previously on sodium fluoride were separately analyzed. In this study etidronate appeared to be an effective treatment for the neurotological symptoms of otosclerosis. In a later study, Brookler (2008) presented two cases of some auditory improvement by the therapy of the bisphosphonates risedronate, etidronate and alendronate. In the two cases described, sodium fluoride and calcium carbonate with supplemental calcium and vitamin D were also prescribed previous to the bisphosphonates treatment. Side effect of the bisphosphonates were not documented in this study. Brookes in 1985 already pointed out that calcium and vitamin-D replacement therapy can result in hearing improvement in cases of otosclerosis. He suggested that vitamin-D deficiency might probably be a factor in the etiology of some cases of otosclerosis and that medications such as fluoride, calcium, or vitamin D may help to slow the hearing loss, but the benefits have not yet been proved. A significant problem of the bisphosphonates treatment is the side effect of possible vitamin-D deficiency and osteomalacia as seen by Boyce *et al.* (1984) in Paget's disease. Furthermore, nausea, dyspepsia or ulceration of the intestines can occur as complication of the therapy; acute renal failure and hypocalcaemia have also been described. Boumans and Poublon (1991) observed in two patients with active stapedial otosclerosis and sensorineural hearing loss who were treated with amino-hydroxy-propylidene bisphosphonate no effect on the Schwartze sign during the following therapy, and no changes in the audiometric data of the patients occurred during a one-year follow up. In both patients a sudden bilateral loss of hearing occurred and it was concluded that this serious deafness was a side effect due to the treatment with amino-hydroxy-propylidene bisphosphonate. Yaşil *et al.* (1998) also described two patients who encountered further hearing loss during oral etidronate treatment for otosclerosis. It must be concluded that bisphosphonate therapy can in potential be ototoxic, although this side effect is very rare. Like the sodium-fluoride therapy, a regular follow up of patients is warranted. Up until now there are no studies available to prove that the use of bisphosphonates interrupt the cochlear otosclerotic process.

2. Alternative well-meant therapies and advices

2.1. Advices

Already in 1908, Tweedie from London described some points in the etiology and the treatment of otosclerosis. He concluded that any surgical and local treatment finally led to an increased deafness.

According to Tweedie it was very important to maintain all the functions of the body in the best possible state. A healthy action of the alimentary tract should be insured and any other concurrent disease like anemia should be treated. To keep the otosclerotic patient in an optimal shape, sufficient exercise, fresh air, judicious clothing and diet were strongly advised. Because worry and burn out were believed to act unfavorably on the course of otosclerosis, avoidance of these stress moments were recommended when possible. Also a limitation of the number of children was suggested, as it could have an influence on the symptoms of the ear disease. In general it was also believed that alcohol and tobacco should be avoided when otosclerosis was diagnosed. Reasons for these advices were unknown. Some authors, like Van Gangelen (1945), believed that a residency at the sea shore was not advised because the sound of the rolling waves could exacerbate tinnitus and furthermore the otosclerosic process. Burger (1956) advised otosclerotic patients to avoid loud or pounding noise, especially in factories. Motorcycling and shooting were also forbidden for those who suffered from otosclerosis. An important advice was that otosclerosis patients should learn lip reading as soon as possible and that in serious cases a hearing aid could be of help. In cases of tinnitus concomitant with otosclerosis, bromine (two to three gr per day), phenobarbital (30-60 mg three times per day) or potassium chloride (300 mg three times per day) were often prescribed. Results of these treatments have not been well documented in literature. Some ear doctors warned that refrain of treatment of otosclerosis could end up in patients turning to quackery (Table 3).

Table 3. Early advices and avoidances in lifestyle for otosclerosis patients.

Advice	Avoidance
Avoid quackery	Alcohol
Fresh air	Loud noise
Healthy life style	Motorcycling
Healthy diet	Overwork
Judicious clothing	Shooting
Limitation of children	The sea shore
Sufficient exercise	Tobacco
	Worry

2.2. Ayurveda and otosclerosis

Ten percent of the population of India suffers from hearing impairment, which is about 100 million people. In India, otosclerosis is more common in the south than it is in the north where its prevalence varies from one to three percent, according to Sabitha *et al.* (1997).

Ayurveda or ayurvedic medicine is a form of alternative traditional medicine from India. Over many centuries, ayurvedic practitioners developed a number of medicinal preparations and surgical procedures for the treatment of various ailments. Ayurveda is based on the use of numerous plant-based medicines and treatments. Often minerals, including sulfur, arsenic, lead, copper sulfate and gold are added. This practice of adding minerals to herbal medicine is known as *rasa shastra*. Because of the relatively high prevalence of otosclerosis in India, the ayurvedic system also has medical treatments for otosclerosis. The ayurvedic treatment for otosclerosis is aimed at the preservation of hearing and attempting to halt or reverse the process of otosclerosis. To prevent damage to the inner ear and the resultant sensorineural hearing loss in otosclerosis, medicines like Kaishor-Guggulu, Tapyadi-Loh, Ekang-Veer-Ras and Bruhat-Vat-Chintamani are used. For the same purpose herbal medicines like Haritaki (*Terminalia chebula*), Amalaki (*Emblica officinalis*), Manjishtha (*Rubia cordifolia*), Saariva (*Hemidesmus indicus*), Punarnava (*Boerhaavia diffusa*), Kutki (*Picrorrhiza kurroa*), Asthishrunkhala (*Cissus quadrangularis*), Laxa (purified wax), Guduchi (*Tinospora cordifolia*) and Musta (*Cyperus rotundus*) can be prescribed. To reverse the process of otosclerosis, the ayurvedic treatment knows medicines like Shankh-Bhasma, Godanti-Bhasma, Praval-Bhasma, Praval-Panchamrut and Panchamrut-Parpati, which can be used in combination with medicines like Tamra-Bhasma, Abhrak-Bhasma and Trivang-Bhasma. Most of these medicines are high-quality herbal extracts in tablet form, which are easy to take. It is claimed that these Ayurveda treatments are effective and safe for long-term use. Through the internet it is easy to get these alternative products nowadays without prescriptions (Valiathan, 2008). However, Saper *et al.* (2008) studied the prevalence of Ayurvedic medicines available through the internet and they discovered that most products contained detectable lead, mercury, or arsenic and that the herbs also contain toxic compounds. In about 20% of these Ayurvedic treatments tested, toxic levels of these heavy metals were found. The quality control of these products is not sufficient. Current practices derived (or reportedly derived) from Ayurvedic medicines are regarded as part of complementary and alternative medicine. Unfortunately, Pubmed and Scophus search machines show no scientific data on the results or the side effects of the medical Ayurveda treatment for otosclerosis.

3. X-ray treatment of otosclerosis

The history of radiation therapy or radiotherapy can be traced back to experiments made soon after the discovery of x-rays. On November 8, 1895, Wilhelm Conrad Röntgen (1845-1923; Fig. 15), Professor of Physics in Würzburg, Germany, discovered by accident an image cast from his cathode ray generator, projected far beyond the possible range of the cathode rays (now known as an electron beam). Further investigation showed that the rays were generated at the point of contact of the cathode ray beam on the interior of the vacuum tube and they penetrated many kinds of matter. It was soon demonstrated that exposure to radiation rays could produce cutaneous burns. Doctors began to

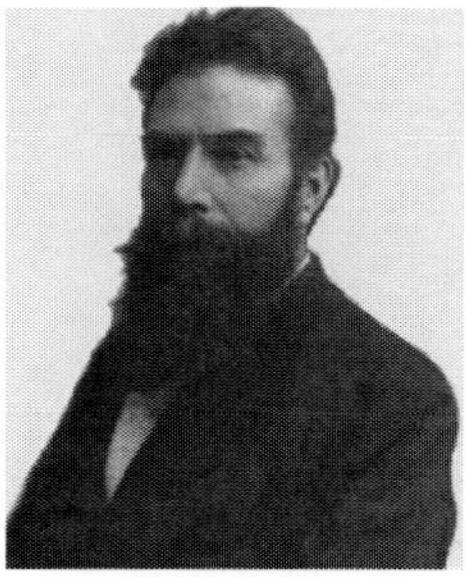

Fig. 15. Wilhelm Conrad Röntgen.

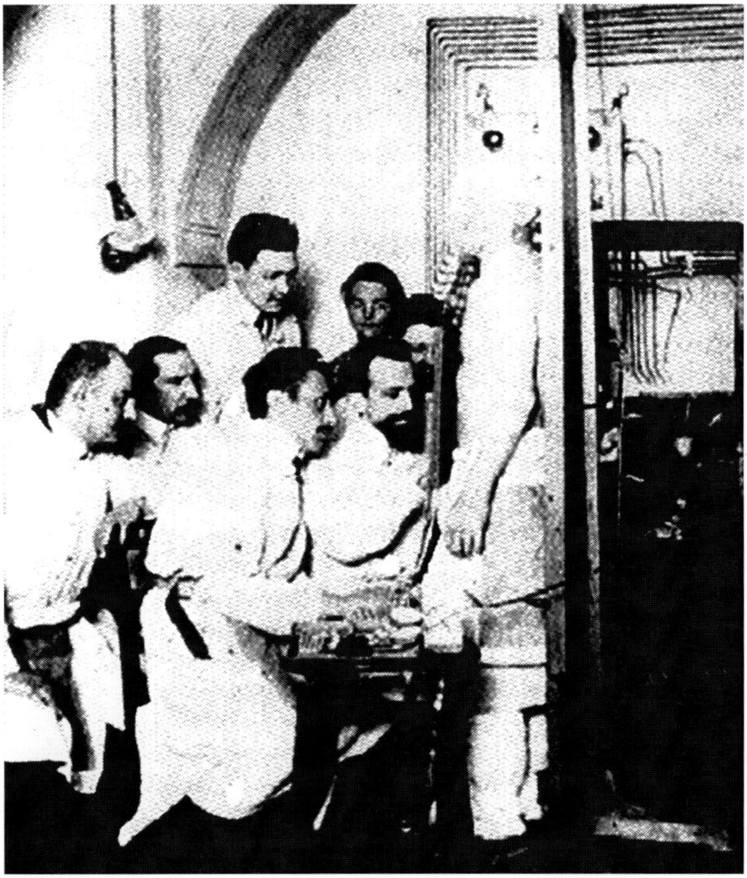

Fig. 16. Gottwald Schwarz (standing), examining a patient.

use radiation to treat growths and lesions produced by diseases such as lupus, rodent ulcer and also later cases of otosclerosis. Radiation was generally believed to have bactericidal properties, so when radium was discovered, in addition to treatments similar to those used with x-rays, it was also used as an additive to medical treatments for diseases such as tuberculosis, where there were resistant bacilli. Because radiation was found to exist in hot spring fountains which were reputed for their curative powers, it was marketed as a wonder cure for all sorts of diseases. It was believed by medical science that small doses of radiation would cause no harm and that harmful effects of large doses were only temporary.

In 1908, Jaulin, a French radiologist, was one of the first scientists who tried to treat middle-ear infections by using X-ray treatment. He used an ear speculum to direct the X-rays to the tympanic membrane. In six out of ten patients treated, hearing improved and the tinnitus diminished.

The famous radiologist from Vienna, Gottwald Schwartz (1880-1959; Fig. 16), a pupil of Holzknecht, started to treat three patients with middle ear affections with X-ray therapy by administering six doses at monthly intervals. In one case (a 16-year-old patient) he observed a surprisingly good hearing result, while in the other cases the hearing did not improve.

Hans Ortloff from Freiburg, together with Kahler and Bloch, started a research on the X-ray treatment of otosclerosis in 1913. For the application of the treatment, the widest possible ear funnel was used. The auricle and the surrounding skin were protected by impenetrable material. The patients were treated in upright position. For the application of the X-ray a special pipe (Müller-Uri) was used, with water cooling. In three days, one third of the normal X-ray treatment was given, which was repeated after two to three weeks. Ten patients (three male and seven female) presenting with hearing loss and tinnitus received the treatment after counseling for otosclerosis. The results of the treatment were negative with respect to the hearing function. In some cases a slight improvement in the tinnitus was observed, but unfortunately the long-term results were return of tinnitus and deafness. (Table 4.)

Table 4. Results of X-ray treatment in otosclerosis by Ortloff 1913.

Case	Sex	Age	Hearing loss since	Ears treated	Result
1	Female	19	10 years	Right ear	Unsuccessful
2	Male	38	10 years	Right ear	Initial improvement, later vertigo
3	Female	25	?	Both ears	?
4	Female	17		Both ears	Unsuccessful - negative
5	Male	34	½ year	Both ears	Initially better, but hearing unchanged
6	Male	23	2 years	Both ears	Hearing unchanged
7	Female	20	Some years	Both ears	Tinnitus gone, but returned after treatment
8	Female	18	3 years	Both ears	Hearing unchanged
9	Female	35	Many years	Both ears	Unsuccessful
10	Female	22	Many years	Both ears	Tinnitus diminished

The conclusion of this study was that the fixation of the stapes in otosclerosis was unchanged after X-ray treatment. Whether the otosclerotic process could be stopped by radiotherapy was unclear but if so, the treatment was believed to be an acquisition. X-ray treatment was considered to be harmless and allegedly promoted the collaboration between otologists and radiologists. Ortloff and his colleagues regretted that they could not get favorable results similar to those published by Jaulin and Schwarz earlier.

In 1921, Douglas Webster, a radiologist from London, remarked that Ortloff probably had been unfortunate in his choice of cases because of the longstanding history (more than ten years) of the otosclerostic complaints. Furthermore he commented on the insufficiently penetrating ray and total dosage used. Webster visited Siebenmann in Basel, Switzerland, who shared with him his views on the theory of X-ray treatment in very severe cases of otosclerosis. In a few cases the results of the treatment were positive in the respect that the usually inevitable progress of the disabling hearing loss was stopped. After his visit to Basel, Webster treated two cases of otosclerosis according to the radiotherapy schedule suggested by Siebenmann. In one case (male patient of 37 years), hearing and tinnitus remained stationary during therapy, without signs of progression of the disease. In the other case (a woman of 25) of hereditary otosclerosis, the X-ray therapy was a success. After three months of treatment the patient could hear the clock in her home again that she had not heard for eight months. Her low-toned tinnitus had almost disappeared. Her hearing was tested later by the ear specialist Dr. Wrigley and a definitive hearing improvement was found. However, in a comment on the publication of Webster in *Lancet*, Harold Barnwell stated that the article was too premature at this early stage and it could raise false hopes among the numerous unfortunate sufferers from otosclerosis. According to Barnwell, the results of X-ray treatment were not very convincing, especially in the early stages of the disease. In 1913, Frey and Kriser, radiologists from Vienna, Austria, reported positive results of their therapeutic treatment with Röntgen rays in cases of otosclerosis and they encouraged the continuation of their treatment. In a discussion in the Klinischer Wochenschrift on this statement, H. Thilemann from Berlin mentioned on the other hand no influence of the Röntgentherapy on the otosclerotic process at all.

Because of the interest of the possible role of cerebral pituitary, the suprarenals, the parathyroids, and the ovaries in an intimate relation to otosclerosis, already mentioned by Sohier Bryant in 1915, Warwick and Stevenson performed a literature study (1926) on an endocrine factor in otosclerosis. They concluded that in otosclerosis a hereditary factor is important and that certain disorders of certain endocrine glands were also the causative factors. In their view, pregnancy led to hypo-functioning of the ovaries and this resulted in hyper-functioning of the pituitary and thyroid, leading to an increased calcium metabolism which was finally responsible for the histological alterations in otosclerosis. In a later study, the same authors, inspired by the work of Richardson (1923) and Frey and Kriser (1924), believed that inhibition of the calcium-increasing glands could be a treatment for otosclerosis. They introduced X-ray application to irradiate the entire thyroid to inhibit the thyroid, and irradiated the temporal bone with the same dosage. Each ovary and its surrounding tissue was then irradiated in the same way. These irradiations were repeated monthly. In the temporal bone irradiation, the rays were guided to the ankylosis of the stapes in the fenestra ovalis with the aim to destroy the cells active in this division. The sella turcica being in the same irradiation field as the temporal bone was considered to be an advantage to inhibit the pituitary gland as well. However, after this publication on local radiation through the ear canal as treatment for progressive otosclerosis, no other studies on this subject have been published in international literature.

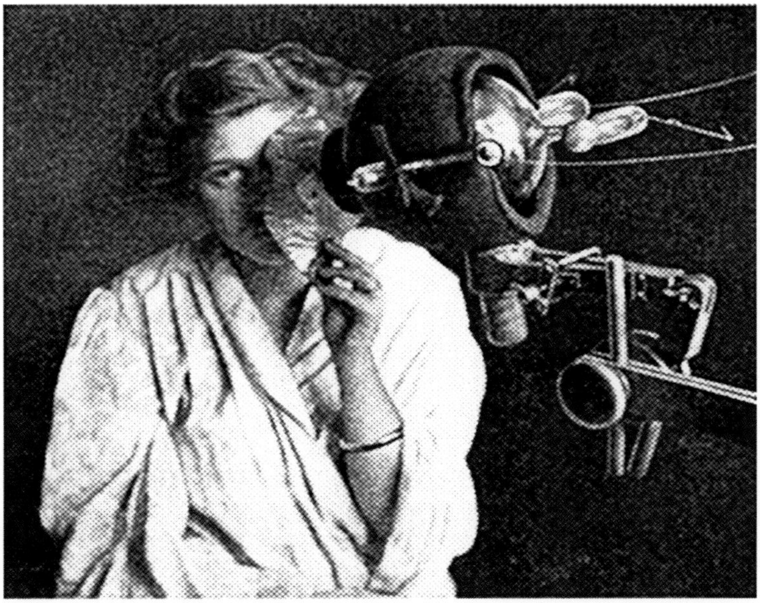

Fig. 17. An example of local treatment with X-rays.

In 1926, Stevenson and Wilson introduced radium treatment of the middle ear and demonstrated preliminary results of two cases of otosclerosis treated successfully with radium therapy. The treatment existed of a radium emanation glass capillary placed within a bronze tube and inserted in the external ear canal close to the drum. The radium capillary was about four mm from the drum. The tube projected from the ear and was held firmly in place at the external meatus by packing with cotton wool, steadied with strapping (Fig. 17). The treatment lasted 24 hours and both ears were treated at the same time. Upon removal of the radium tube, some injection was observed in the meatus or tympanum. The results of this treatment were promising for middle-ear infections as for otosclerosis; it seemed that the treatment did not progress the process and in fact the authors hoped the disease had been arrested. In their discussion they pointed out that in these cases systematical re-education of the auditory brain centers was absolutely essential, for example by means of the Zünd-Burguet electrophonoïde, which produces sounds similar to those of the human voice. Given the preliminary increase in the functioning power of the conducting apparatus by means of radium, this apparatus should give excellent results. Stevenson and Wilson believed that if the improvement they found was permanent, and could be repeated in other cases, a tremendous advance was made, and radium therapy would gain a permanent position in the treatment of this distressing condition of otosclerosis. However, radium therapy has never been introduced as a successful treatment for otosclerosis.

The widespread use of radium X-rays in medicine ended when it was discovered that physical tolerance was lower than expected and exposure caused long-term cell damage that could result in carcinoma up to 40 years after treatment. The use of radiation continues today as a treatment for cancer, where it is applied with strict safety precautions.

4. Re-education machines

Re-education of the deaf and patients with hearing impairment by means of sounds regulated so as to stimulate and awaken the dormant sense of hearing from physiological apathy was the basis for the development of instruments and devices to treat hearing loss. The devices were designed after the example of the early oto-massage apparatus developed by Delstanche and Breitung.

4.1. Kinésiphone

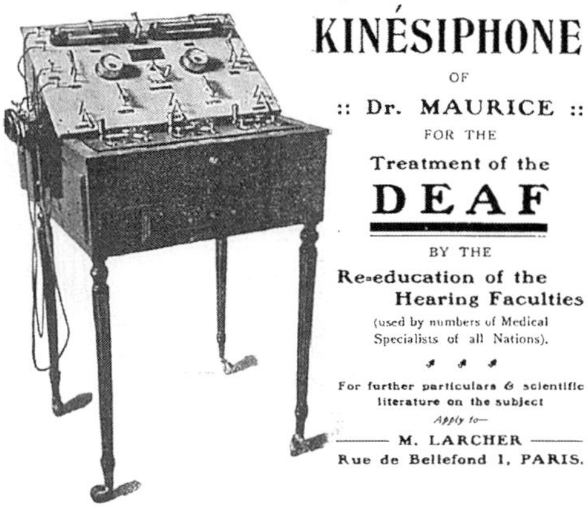

Fig. 18. Maurice's Kinésiphone.

In 1912, Dr. A. Maurice from Paris constructed an apparatus which he called the Kinésiphone (Fig. 18), for auditive re-education. The Kinésiphone produced sonorous vibrations, similar to those of the human voice, in all frequencies between 80 and 3,500 cycles of all of the vocal sounds. The sounds, of variable intensity, were delivered to the ear by headphones. The patient held the vibrating membranes, which were mounted on handles resembling telephone ear-pieces, to his ear. The intensity was increased steadily to the point of tickle but not of pain. The treatment sittings were from six to ten minutes daily and had to be continued for at least fifty times. The Kinésiphone worked by a six-volt accumulator and was furnished with an ammeter to show the amount of current, a voltmeter to test the condition of the accumulator and an interrupter to cut off the current if necessary. In certain cases this was supplemented by diathermy. Maurice believed that it was possible to treat deafness and middle-ear diseases like otosclerosis if only the patient and the doctor had perseverance and believed in the treatment. It was impossible to predict which cases could be improved. He considered therapeutic success to be at least a ten-fold increase in hearing distance. He showed statistically that 75% of the cases were successful; 20% were semi-successful, and

5% were failures. Maurice claimed also that tinnitus and other discomforts concerning the ear condition would be relieved or even disappear after this treatment. In October 1912, a review by D. McKenzie on the Kinésiphone was published in which he criticized the absence of several criteria of testing the hearing during and after treatment. McKenzie noted that tuning-fork tests were needed. The speech and whisper tests had not been done by a second, preferably unbiased observer, and detailed results of the examination of the membrane and of politzerisation were missing. McKenzie hoped that further development of Maurice's treatment device would enhance the results of the Kinésiphone.

H. Lavrand from Lille, also being skeptical about auditory re-education, treated some patients with intractable hearing loss with the Kinésiphone. He only applied the treatment after all usual classic methods had failed. Five cases were described and they showed encouraging results. Although there was no alteration in their hearing, a slight improvement under phonatory massage was achieved. Lavrand (1913) concluded that the Kinésiphone treatment constituted a real progress compared with the existing methods of treatment. It was believed that the re-education device increased the hearing power when other means of treatment did failed. However, the success of the Zünd-Burguet electrophonoïd would soon make the Kinésiphone disappear from the market.

4.2. Zünd-Burguet electrophonoïd

Based upon the idea of re-education of the auditive system using tuning forks and an oral method, Alphonse Zünd-Burguet from Paris developed an device which he called the electrophonoïd. The purpose of the device was massaging the middle-ear structures by using sound waves. The apparatus used notes from the lowest to the highest range – depending on the hearing impairment – which were forced through the middle ear structures. The treatment was arranged so that after the auditory capacity had been determined, the patient heard the complete range from bass to treble. The treatment was started carefully with an increase in intensity toward the end of the session. The Zünd-Burguet electrophonoïd was rather popular in the treatment of deafness and 'sclerosis'. Zünd-Burguet wrote a book in which he explaned his theories and his treatment (Fig. 19). Raoult studied the results of 35 patients (13 were patients of Zünd-Burguet) who were treated with the electrophonoïd device. In the majority of these cases the improvement in hearing maintained. The sooner the complaint was treated, the better the results and the prognosis for the ear disease.

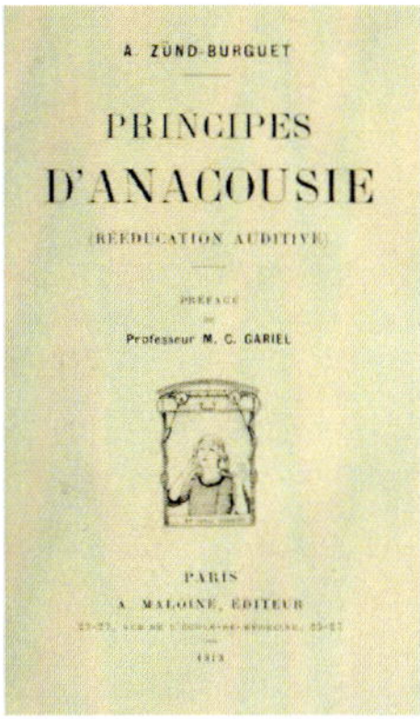

Fig. 19. Alphonse Zünd-Burguet's book explaining the auditive re-education (1913).

In 1914, Hubby from New York thought that all hearing impairments could always be expected to show a certain improvement after treatment with the Zünd-Burguet method. He had treated over 20 cases of otosclerosis, during 50 sessions each. In most cases, hearing was at least ten times better after treatment.

Later, Macleod Yearsley reported the results of Zünd-Burguet therapy in 200 cases. He had used the treatment since 1925 successfully on 77.5% of the patients. The Zünd-Burguet therapy was said to be especially fit for cases of recent deafness and for children. The distance at which they were able to understand a conversation had increased from a few inches to 4.5 feet. These results remained four to five years. It was believed that the results of the electrophonoïd were due to the vibrating massage, which caused hyperemia in the ear tissues and restored the circulation, thereby influencing the 'sclerotic process'. In a reaction to a statement of Barwell that the results of the Zünd-Burguet treatment appeared to be evancescent, Yearsley referred to his more than ten years experience with the electrophonoïd.

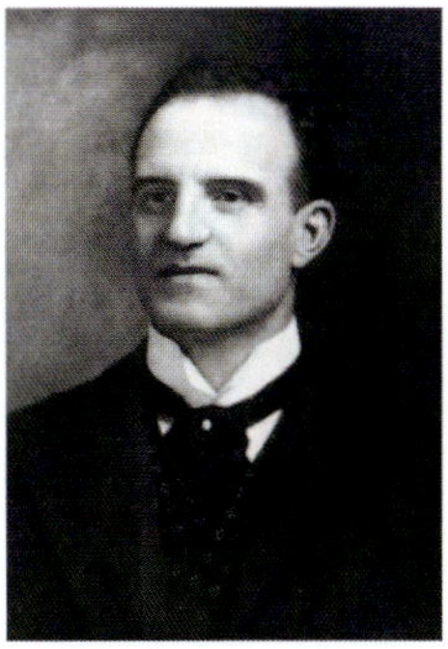

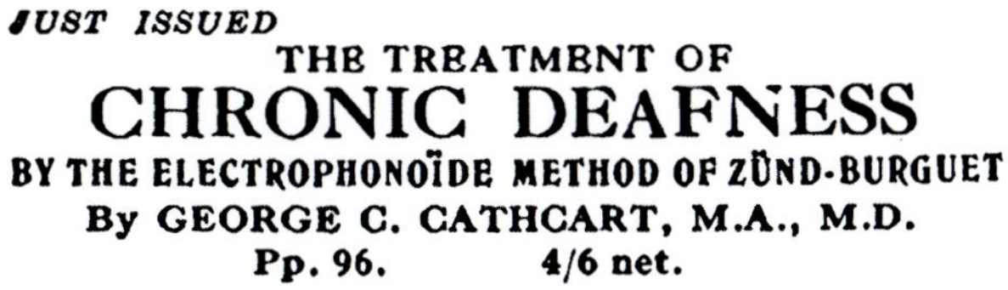

Fig. 20a (above). George Cathart
Courtesy Jean-Paul Wayenborgh

Fig. 20b (left). Advertisement of Cathcart promoting his experience with the Zünd-Burguet electrophonoïd (1926).

George Cathcart (Oxford, UK) re-introduced the electrophonoïd in 1926 (Fig. 20). He underlined the importance of a magneto-electrical device for re-educating the hearing and he pleaded for a good use of the Zünd-Burguet electrophonoïd. Cathcart offered an educative technique by means of a complicated instrument, the electrophone of Zünd-Burguet, which reproduced sound vibrations in the whole range of the human voice, thus giving the necessary physiologic stimulus to the ear. His first studies on treatment with the Zünd-Bruguet electrophonoïd for otosclerosis existed of 97 cases (75 males and 22 females). In 39 of the female patients and 13 of the males deafness had deminished, a success rate of 53.6%. In 1931, Cathcart had treated over 665 cases, including nerve deafness, with an improvement of 73.8%. He had experience with 217 cases of otosclerosis and reported an improvement of 53.9%. In 230 cases of tinnitus an improvement of 68.7% was obtained. He concluded that it was justified to apply the instrument if other surgeons could do one-half as well as he did. Stevenson and Wilson (1926) supported the use of the Zünd-Burguet electrophonoïd as a complement to their radium therapy for otosclerosis.

On May 3, 1935, at the Section of Otology of the Royal Society of Medicine, A. Gray stated that he never had seen any satisfactory results from the Zünd-Burguet method of treatment. Gray defended his treatment with thyroxine locally on the mastoid as an alternative. At that same meeting, J.F. O'Malley mentioned his treatment by local application of heat on the otosclerotic ear. He had made an asbestos-lined box, designed to include the whole mastoid and ear, the rest of the head being shut off from the heating apparatus. He had tried this in twenty cases over a period of one year. The results were not convincing and he had stopped the treatment.

Having seen Cathcart using the Zünd-Burguet electrophonoïd vibromassage, aural surgeon J.A. Keen from Leicester (1932) started to apply the treatment in cases of the Ménière syndrome and observed that the vibromassage was especially useful in cases of Ménière attacks. Only one paper appeared on this subject.

In 1933, O. Voss and his engineer M. Mülwert developed a device similar to the Zünd-Burguet electrophonoïd, with the main difference that Mülwert's device used high-frequency sound waves which were beyond the range of hearing. This device was also used and tested in cases of otosclerosis. J. Schmalix (1950) observed that all otosclerosis patients who had been treated with ultrasound complained of dizziness after the treatment. He concluded that ultrasound affected the inner ear in a negative way and that because there was no improvement after the treatment, ultrasound was contra-indicated for otosclerosis. Z. Angeluscheff and L.L. Coleman (1953) performed histological studies on ultrasonics and the bone changes that occur after experimental treatment. They suggested that just ultrasonic vibrations could be an etiological factor to the onset of otosclerosis. Treatment of otosclerosis by re-education machines like the electrophonoïd vibromassage, the kinésiphone or the ultrasonic device became obsolete after the success of fenestration surgery.

5. Hearing aids and otosclerosis

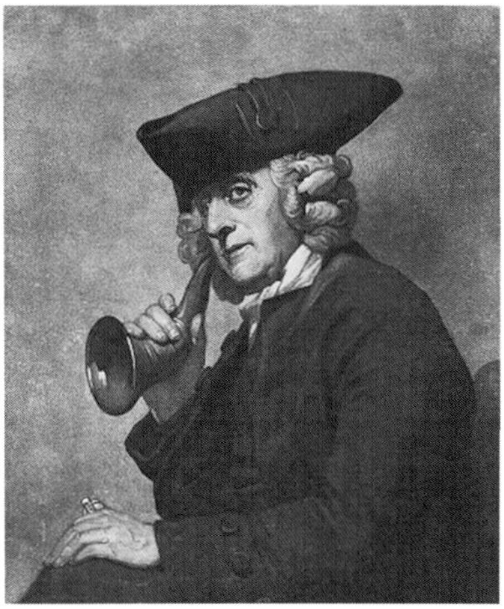

Fig. 21. The ear trumpet in the golden age.

Long before the disease otosclerosis was known, the only treatment for hearing loss was the ear trumpet (Fig. 21). Ear trumpets were popular and became more effective during the 1800s. The length and shape of the horn-like devices determined their effectiveness in transmitting sound. Probably the first hearing aids for otosclerosis were the bone-conduction teeth stimulators developed by R.S. Rhodes (1879) and T.W. Graydon (1880). Otosclerosis being a bone-conducting disease these fans were an acceptable help in hearing rehabilitation. The Audiphone of Rhodes (Fig. 22) and the Dentaphone of Graydon (Figs. 23-25) conveyed sound to the inner ear through the teeth. The user held the bone conduction fan in his hand and a small wooden mouthpiece was held tightly between the teeth. Sound was picked up by the diaphragm, and was passed to the user's teeth via vibrations through a piece of silk-covered wire. The fan provided a benefit of up to 30 dB, a gain comparable to listening to someone speaking from a distance of two feet

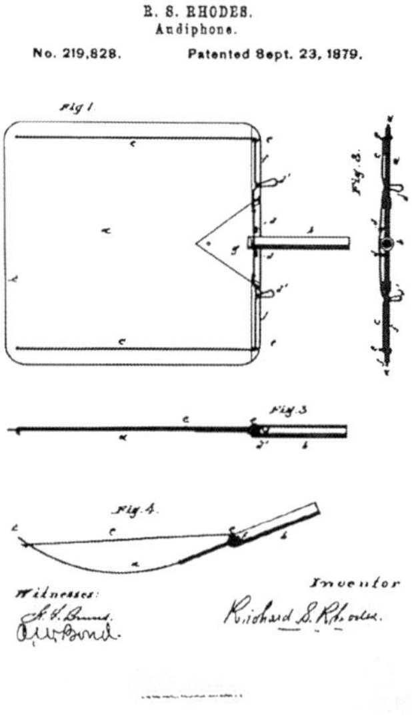

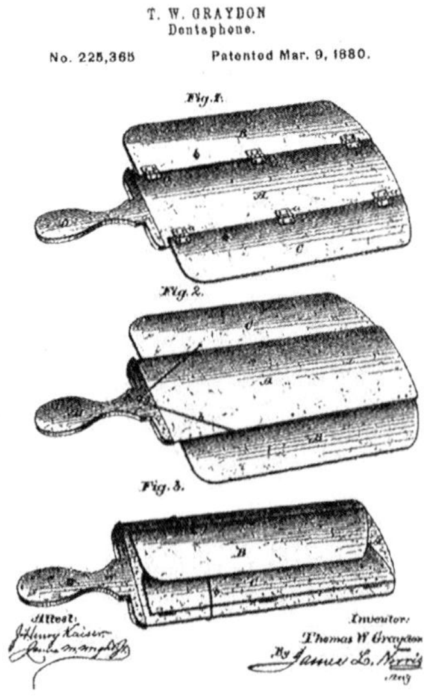

Fig. 22 (left). Rhodes' Audiphone.

Fig. 23 (right). Graydon's Dentaphone.

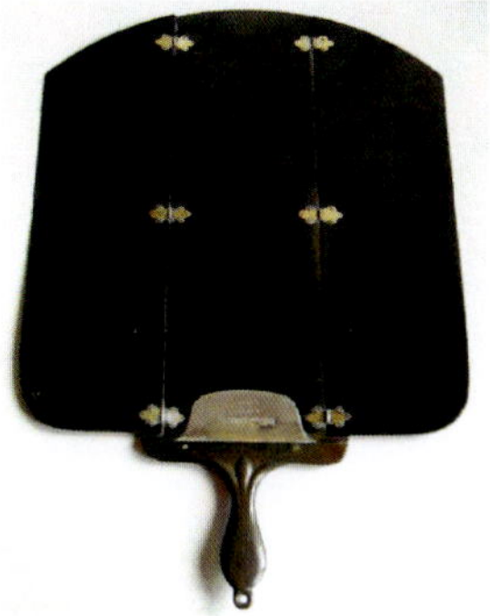

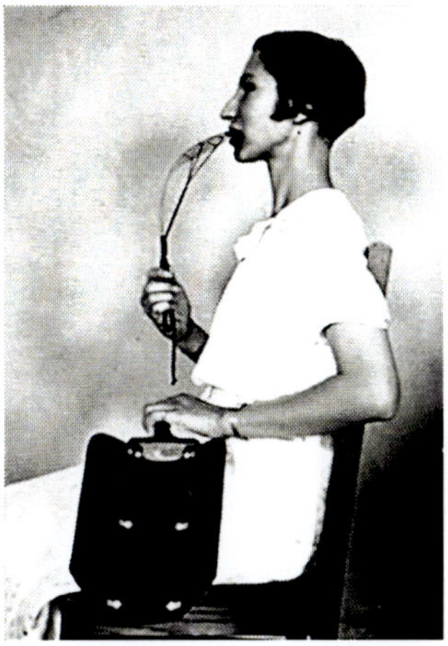

Fig. 24 (left). The Dentaphone.

Fig. 25 (right). The Dentaphone in action.

rather than sixty-four feet. The fan also provided hearing rehabilitation; furthermore, it could also help to diagnose whether the hearing loss was of bone-conducting origin. Although the Audiphone of Rhodes was awarded with a medal at the World's Columbian Exhibition in 1893 in Chicago, the success of these bone-conduction teeth stimulators for otosclerosis patients seems to be doubtful. There is no literature available on this treatment for hearing loss in otosclerosis.

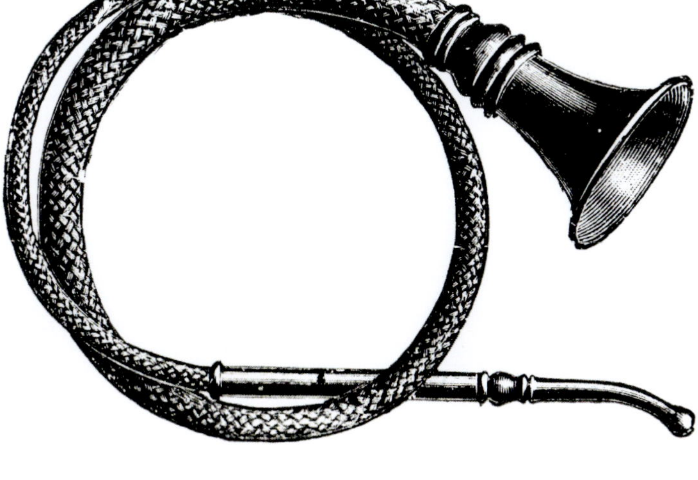

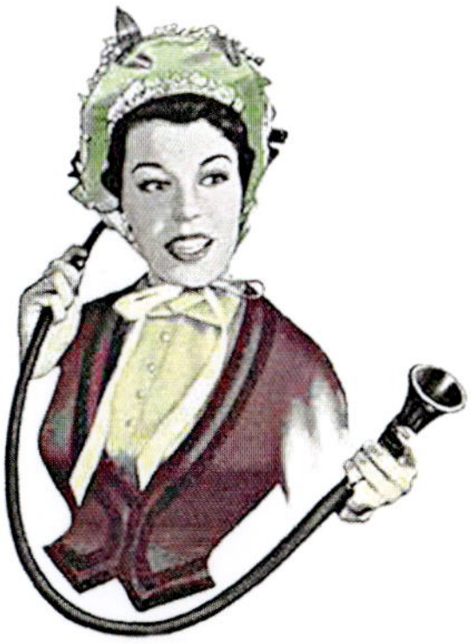

Fig. 26 (left). Dunker's hearing tube.

Fig. 27 (right). A happy user of the Dunkers hearing tube.

In his textbook of 1905, G. Brühl (in cooperation with A. Politzer) does not mention the existence of the bone-conduction teeth stimulators anymore. At that time, the so-called Dunkersche Horschlauch was considered to be the most important hearing aid (Figs. 26 & 27). This hearing device consisted of a bendable tube of one meter length and two to three centimeters in diameter, with on one side an earpiece and on the other side a funnel for the reception of sound. The hearing tube only facilitated the conversation between the otosclerotic patient and other persons, it did not work well in traffic or at social events.

In 1914, O. Körner still recommended Dunker's hearing tube as hearing aid of choice. He also recommended lip-reading lessons for the treatment of patients with otosclerosis. Körner was critical about the electrical hearing apparatus that had just been introduced. He warned against the damage these hearing aids could cause and more specifically the risk of tinnitus. G.J. Jenkins and colleagues (1914) advised against any instrumental hearing device in the earliest stage of otosclerosis. In their opinion, when the patient reached a degree that he could not hear a speaker in a hall but still could have an ordinary conversation, the use of a 'trumpet' was recommended, and only beyond that stage, a carefully selected hearing device combined with lip reading could be an option.

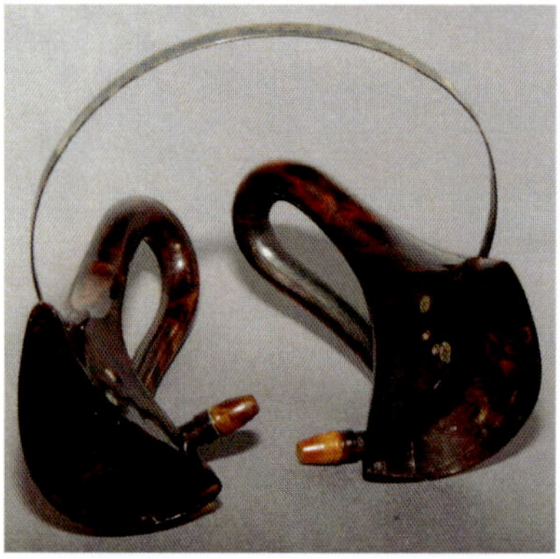

Fig. 28. Auricles.

Jenkins was a great advocate of the so-called auricles (Fig. 28) as hearing aid in cases of otosclerosis. He felt that since the electrical hearing instruments were so much advocated, these auricles were rather neglected. He also stated that the auricle was more useful than electrical instruments in cases of marked inner-ear deafness. The auricle was very suitable for women as it could simply be hidden in long hair. Because of the evolution of the electrical technology at the beginning of the twentieth century, the popularity of auricles, trumpets and speaking tubes as hearing aids rapidly decreased. The first electric hearing aids were large and impractical desktop devices, but as technology improved, their components became smaller. After transistors were introduced, hearing aids even became portable.

Electrical instruments for the treatment of hearing loss are now known as conventional hearing aids. Although they can play an important role in the rehabilitation of hearing and also in otosclerosis, only a few publications on the subject are available, which is probably due to the great success of the stapes surgery as introduced by Shea in 1956. Because of the negative points of conventional hearing aids and the very small number of complications of stapedectomy, patients prefer stapes surgery over hearing aids. Also, otolaryngology consultants in the UK offer the use of a hearing aid as an option for the treatment of otosclerosis in only 2.8% of cases, according to a survey from Raut *et al.* (2002). In his forty-year review of stapes surgery for otosclerosis, Shea demonstrated that 30 years after a successful stapedectomy about 30% of the cases do need the help of a conventional hearing aid.

Smyth and Hassard demonstrated that after a successful stapedectomy on average most of the patients require a conventional hearing aid after 13 years post-operatively and that after a stapedotomy a hearing aid was needed after 21 years of this type of surgery post-operatively.

Lundman *et al.* (1999) studied 95 patients operated unilaterally for otosclerosis and he observed, besides tinnitus, dizziness and sound-distortion, that in 18% of these cases the patients needed a hearing aid after three to eight years after the operation. Tange and Grolman (2009) demonstrated that in a post-operative follow up of 10 to 21 years after stapes surgery the reconstruction with a stapes prosthesis remained stable, but that the cochlear function diminished during the same period. It is important to inform patients about this phenomenon in an informed consent. Recently Redfors and Möller (2011) finished a 30-year follow-up study on otosclerosis and stapes surgery (65 patients) and observed that in 66% of cases a moderate to profound hearing loss occurred. They concluded that in the long run almost all patients with otosclerosis need audiological rehabilitation and hearing aids after all. This statement is certainly true for cases of far-advanced otosclerosis involving the inner ear. Unfortunately, suitable comparative studies between hearing aids for mixed-type and sensorineural otosclerosis and surgical outcomes are not available yet. Nevertheless, hearing aids will play an important role in the treatment of otosclerosis as a result of aging, even after successful stapes surgery.

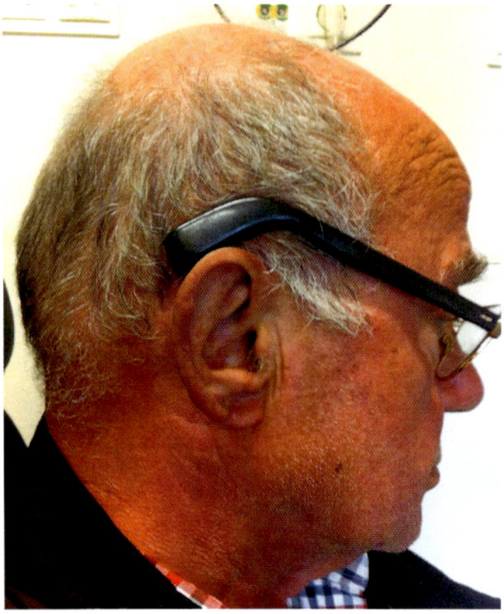

Fig. 29. A pair of glasses with integrated bone conductor.

After the bone-conduction teeth stimulator, the carbon microphone was developed, allowing the construction of the bone-conduction vibrator which was placed on the mastoid area. In the newer versions of the bone-conduction vibrator, the vibrator was integrated into a pair of glasses (Fig. 29).

This device could be a solution for the treatment of conduction hearing loss in similar cases of otosclerosis, but was applied more in cases of a radical cavity and chronic running ears. In 1981, Tjellstrom and co-workers developed the idea to implant a titanium vibrator into the mastoid bone and through the skin as a hearing aid in cases of conduction hearing loss, to overcome the skin problems that occurred with the classic bone-conduction aids. These bone-anchored hearing aids (BAHA; Figs. 30-32) have since been an alternative treatment in some cases of otosclerosis. In cases of difficulties in using a conventional hearing aid, like chronic external otitis in an only hearing ear with otosclerosis, the BAHA could be considered a surgical solution for hearing rehabilitation. According the data from Wazen *et al.* (2008), in only 4.8% of cases where a BAHA was indicated the etiology of the hearing loss was otosclerosis. Besides the conventional hearing aids, the bone-anchored hearing aids may offer a low-risk alternative to stapes surgery for otosclerosis, but in about 10% of the cases skin problems can be a serious side effect.

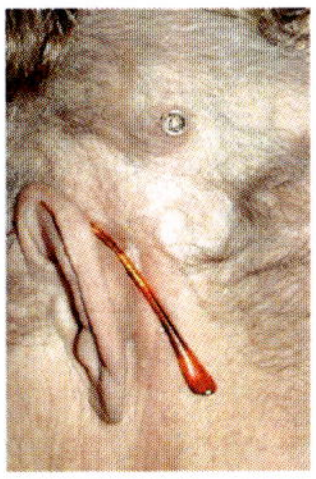

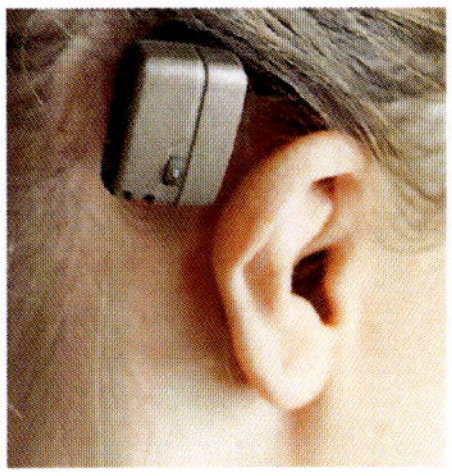

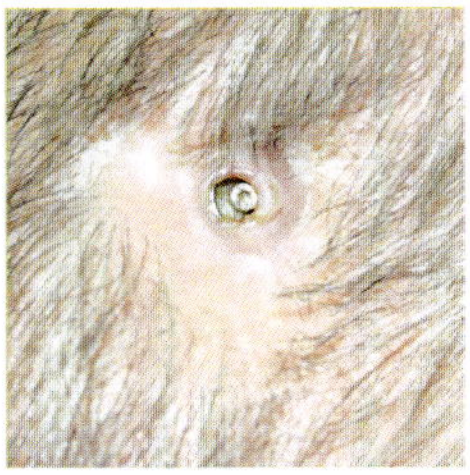

Fig. 30 (left). A BAHA abutment on the skull.

Fig. 31 (middle). A BAHA processor in position.

Fig. 32 (right). Overgrowth of skin over the BAHA abutment as side effect.

Chapter three

Treatment of otosclerosis and pregnancy

1. Pregnancy and otosclerosis

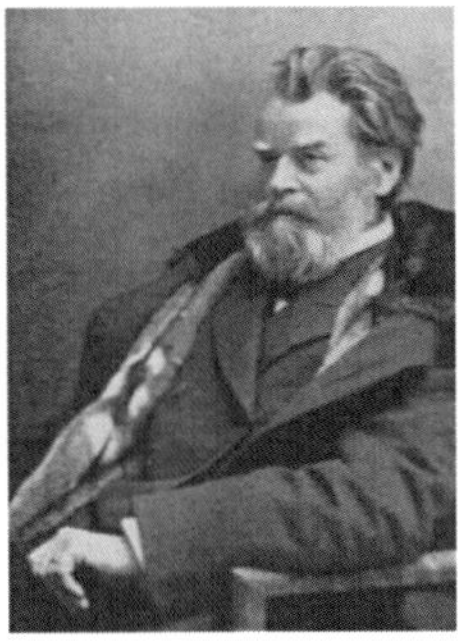

Fig. 33. Friedrich Bezold.

Otosclerosis occurs more often in females than in males. Friedrich Bezold (1842-1908; Fig. 33) calculated the percentage of females and males affected by otosclerosis in a retrospective study over the period 1884-1892. He found that 60.2-61.1% females and 41.8-58.2% males were affected.

Heimann (1909) stated that the disease occurred twice as much in women than in men. Wolf (1895) observed the influence of pregnancy on the hearing organ. Sohier Bryant mentioned that possibly pregnancy or the puerperium intoxicated the temporal bone. The temporal bone might be affected by bone changes

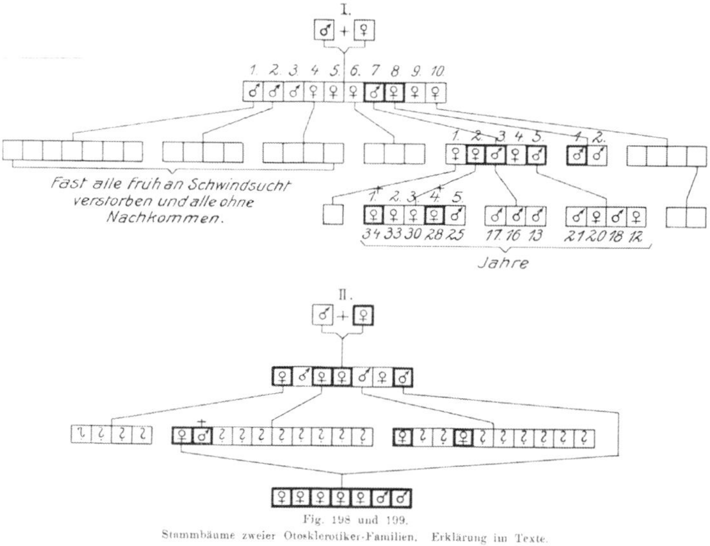

Fig. 34. Pedigree of an otosclerotic family studied by Körner 1914.

which occurred in the puerperium, thus causing otosclerosis. Politzer was one of the first to suggest there was a relation between otosclerosis and puerperium and that otosclerosis was a true infective puerperal osteitis. In 1904, Denker pointed out the possible relation between otosclerosis and pregnancy and the puerperium. He suggested that in cases of a strong hereditary pathway of otosclerosis, the female patient should consider prevention of conception.

During one of the meetings of the German otological society, Denker describes the sad side of pregnant otosclerotic patients with a rapid loss of hearing and severe tinnitus. Körner (1914) described the observation that the loss of hearing in otosclerosis is usually a slow process, but in pregnancy this loss is often very progressive. He was rather extreme in his thoughts on how to advise young girls who were suffering from hearing loss due to otosclerosis. He advised them not to marry or to have children because every pregnancy could create latent determinants. This advice had already been suggested by Tweedie in 1908.

2. Eugenics and otosclerosis

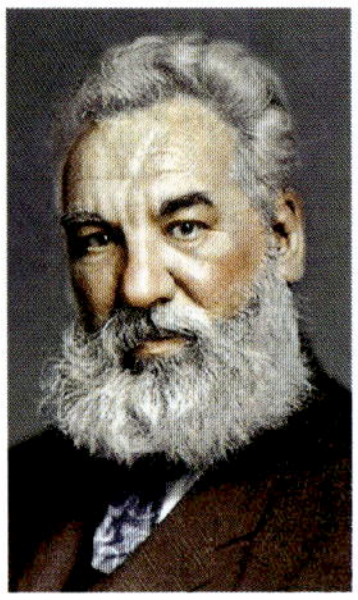
Fig. 35. Alexander Graham Bell.

These ideas of Tweedie and Körner were not new at that time. Already in 1881, the inventor of the telephone Alexander Graham Bell (1847-1922; Fig. 35), investigated the rate of deafness at Martha's Vineyard in Massachusetts.

He noticed that on this island on the East Coast of the United States a high rate of hereditary deafness occurred. The deaf islanders probably were originally immigrants from Weald in the county Kent in England, where hereditary deafness was known in the seventeenth century. The islanders even developed their own language amongst the deaf population. Of all marriages on the island in the late 19th century, 65% were mixed marriages between deaf and hearing, while on the mainland this was 20%. From this Bell concluded that deafness was hereditary in nature and, through noting that congenitally deaf parents were more likely to produce deaf children, tentatively suggested that deaf couples should not marry. In his lecture 'Memoir upon the formation of a deaf variety of the human race' presented by Bell to the National Academy of Sciences on November 13, 1883, he defended his theory. Alexander Graham Bell was one of the earliest modern representatives of eugenics. Eugenics is the science and the social movement which advocated the use of practices aimed at improving the genetic composition of the human race. The basic principles of this movement were certain interpretations of the work on genetics by Gregor Johann Mendel (1822-1884; Fig. 36).

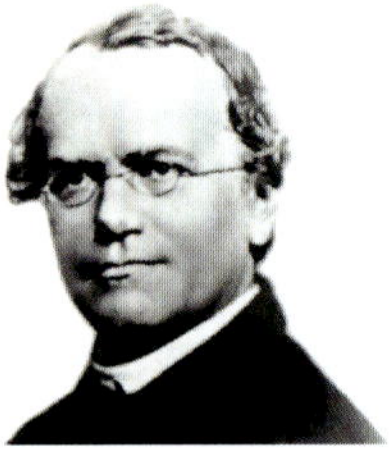
Fig. 36. Gregor Johann Mendel.

Eugenics was widely popular in the early decades of the twentieth century. The biologist Charles Benedict Davenport (1866-1944; Fig. 37) was one of the first scientists to introduce the concepts of Mendelian genetics in the United States and later on worldwide. After receiving a grant of 500.000 dollars of the heirs of the rail-road magnate Edward Henry Harriman, Davenport founded a research centre called the Eugenics Records Office (ERO) in

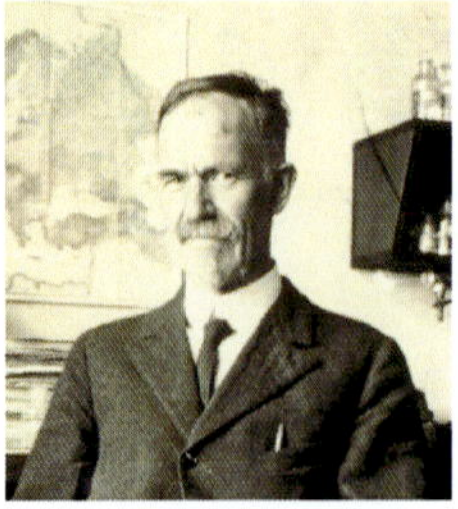
Fig. 37. Charles Benedict Davenport.

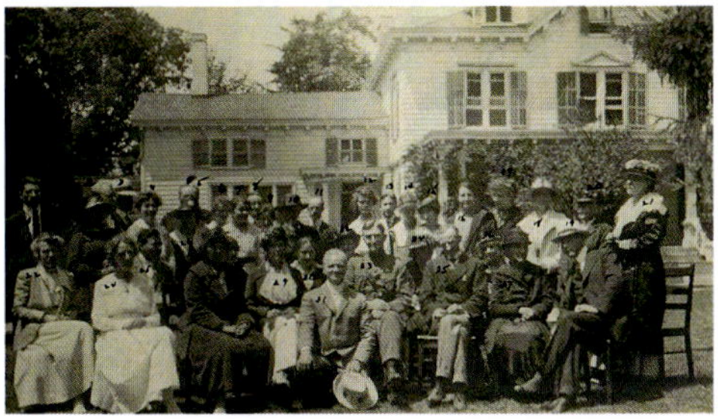

Fig. 38. A summer meeting of the ERO in 1918.

Cold Spring Harbor, USA in 1910 (Fig. 38). Davenport and Harry H. Laughlin (Fig. 39), the later director of ERO, organized three International Congresses on Eugenics. Davenport studied the genetics of different diseases including neurofibromatosis, epilepsy, goiter and otosclerosis and published a book and an article about the heredity of otosclerosis. At the ERO, over 750.000 data were collected and documented about all kinds of genetic diseases and based on these data, Laughlin prepared a voluminous book with the solution to racial betterment. *Eugenical Sterilization in the United States* with a model eugenical sterilization law was published in 1922 (Fig. 40) and provided the scientific basis for later eugenic policies, such as enforced sterilization.

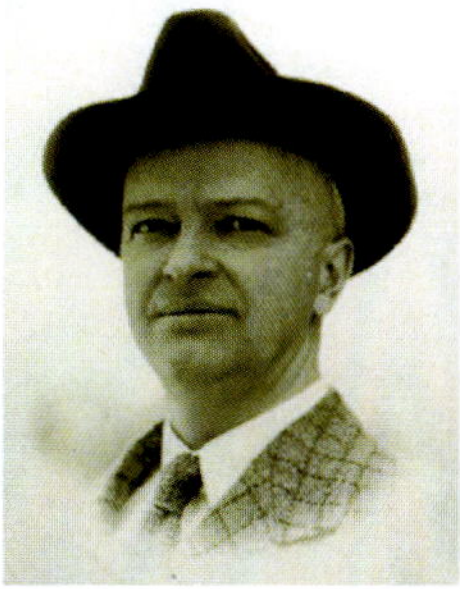

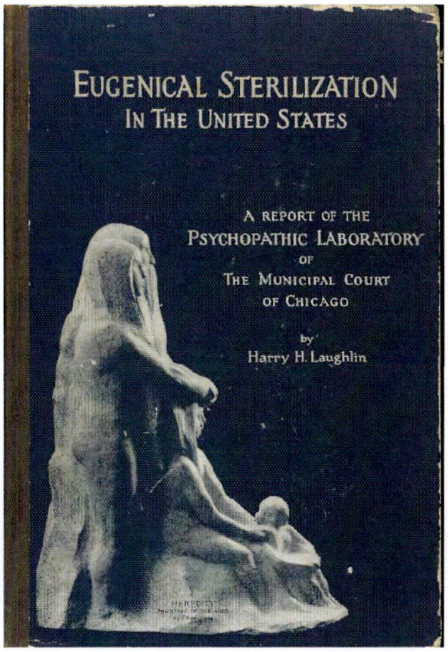

Fig. 39 (left). Harry Hamilton Laughlin (1880-1943).

Fig. 40 (right). The book by Laughlin, published in 1922.

The eugenical sterilizaton law came into force in 1924 in 18 states of the USA. Besides other illnesses and alcoholism, people suffering from deafness (including those with seriously impaired hearing) were included as subjects for eugenic sterilization (Fig. 41) and also, on page 375 of Laughlin's book, otosclerosis is indicated as a hereditary disease eligible for eugenical sterilization.

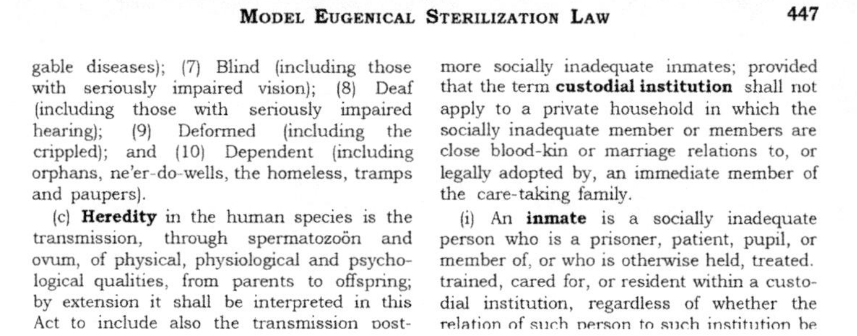

MODEL EUGENICAL STERILIZATION LAW 447

gable diseases); (7) Blind (including those with seriously impaired vision); (8) Deaf (including those with seriously impaired hearing); (9) Deformed (including the crippled); and (10) Dependent (including orphans, ne'er-do-wells, the homeless, tramps and paupers).

(c) **Heredity** in the human species is the transmission, through spermatozoön and ovum, of physical, physiological and psychological qualities, from parents to offspring; by extension it shall be interpreted in this Act to include also the transmission post-

more socially inadequate inmates; provided that the term **custodial institution** shall not apply to a private household in which the socially inadequate member or members are close blood-kin or marriage relations to, or legally adopted by, an immediate member of the care-taking family.

(i) An **inmate** is a socially inadequate person who is a prisoner, patient, pupil, or member of, or who is otherwise held, treated, trained, cared for, or resident within a custodial institution, regardless of whether the relation of such person to such institution be

Fig. 41. Indication # 8 for eugenical sterilization according to Laughlin.

3. Sterilization and artificial abortus and otosclerosis

Artur Blohmke, assistant at the University Earclinic in Königberg, Germany performed in 1918 an extensive study on pregnancy and the etiology and treatment of otosclerosis. He did a survey at different German ear clinics on the question whether pregnancy indeed causes deterioration of hearing in otosclerosis and if in special cases an interruption of the pregnancy was indicated to stop the process of hearing loss. Blohmke received many case reports on hearing loss and severe tinnitus due to pregnancy. He concluded that there was no absolute indication for induced abortus in cases of severe hearing loss and tinnitus in pregnancy with otosclerosis. On the other hand, in pregnancy cases with a tendency to suicide because of severe tinnitus and strong hearing loss, abortion was sometimes performed. Brickner believed (1911) that only interruption of the pregnancy could stop the acute deterioration of hearing and that after the abortion the question of sterilization of the female should be considered. According to Blohmke's survey study, Welty performed at least six abortions between 1910 and 1915 because he believed that there was no other treatment to stop otosclerotic hearing loss due to pregnancy.

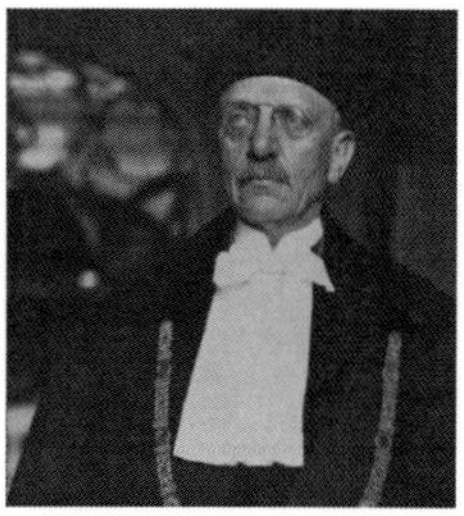
Fig. 42. Hendrik Burger.

Hendrik Burger (1864-1957; Fig. 42) from Amsterdam (known for his comment on otosclerosis: 'Girls after marriage, women after pregnancy') described the dilemma of a case of a pregnant otosclerotic woman in 1923. He did not have much experience with abortion treatment for acute hearing loss during pregnancy, but after careful consideration and following the wish of the female to do everything to save her hearing, Burger decided to interrupt the pregnancy. The patient was a musician and her husband already had children from a previous marriage. The result of the treatment was no progression of the hearing loss. It seemed that the hearing had improved a little and the tinnitus had almost disappeared. Burger concluded his French publication of this case with the comment that a brother of the patient visited him later with the same hearing loss due to otosclerosis, proving the hereditary character of the disease.

At the Third International Eugenics Congress (1932) in New York, presided by Charles Davenport, it was emphasized that birth selection rather than birth control was the method to better the offspring and to rid society of 'the unfit'. He predicted doom of our civilization, unless eugenic measures like compulsory sterilization or even abortion were implemented. Harry Laughlin, director of the ERO, already made recommendations for eugenical sterilization in 1922. In 1933, the German Ernst Rüdin (1874-1952), president of the International Federation of Eugenics Societies, wrote for the Nazi's the 'Gesetz zur Verhütung erbkranken Nachwuchses – GezVeN' or 'Sterilization Law' which was a modification of the model law by Laughlin. Three years later (1936), Laughlin was awarded an honorary degree by the University of Heidelberg for his achievements in the field of the 'science of racial cleansing' at the 550 anniversary of that university. Laughlin never made it to Germany; the State Department advised him not to go to Germany, and he was also involved in a car accident which forced him to stay in the USA.

The 'Sterilization Law' (Fig. 43) in Nazi Germany entered into force in January 1934 by approval of the 'Chancellor of the Reich', Adolf Hitler. This allowed the compulsory sterilization of any citizen who in the opinion of the 'Genetic Health Court' (Erbgesundheitsgericht) suffered from one or more of the – alleged – genetic disorders mentioned on their list. According to this law, a person suffering from any one of the following diseases was considered as hereditary diseased:

1. Congenital mental deficiency,
2. Schizophrenia,
3. Manic-depressive insanity,
4. Hereditary epilepsy,
5. Hereditary chorea (Huntington's disease),

6. Hereditary blindness,
7. Hereditary deafness,
8. Any severe hereditary deformity.

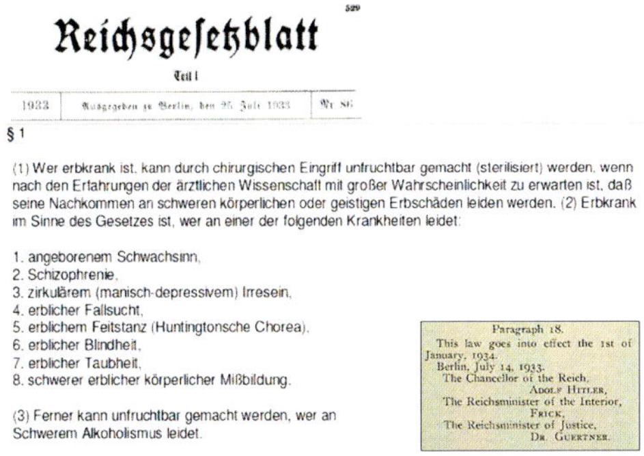

Reichsgesetzblatt 529

Teil I

1933 | Ausgegeben zu Berlin, den 25. Juli 1933 | Nr. 86

§ 1

(1) Wer erbkrank ist, kann durch chirurgischen Eingriff unfruchtbar gemacht (sterilisiert) werden, wenn nach den Erfahrungen der ärztlichen Wissenschaft mit großer Wahrscheinlichkeit zu erwarten ist, daß seine Nachkommen an schweren körperlichen oder geistigen Erbschäden leiden werden. (2) Erbkrank im Sinne des Gesetzes ist, wer an einer der folgenden Krankheiten leidet:

1. angeborenem Schwachsinn,
2. Schizophrenie,
3. zirkulärem (manisch-depressivem) Irresein,
4. erblicher Fallsucht,
5. erblichem Feitstanz (Huntingtonsche Chorea),
6. erblicher Blindheit,
7. erblicher Taubheit,
8. schwerer erblicher körperlicher Mißbildung.

(3) Ferner kann unfruchtbar gemacht werden, wer an Schwerem Alkoholismus leidet.

Paragraph 18.
This law goes into effect the 1st of January, 1934.
Berlin, July 14, 1933.
The Chancellor of the Reich,
Adolf Hitler,
The Reichsminister of the Interior,
Frick,
The Reichsminister of Justice,
Dr. Guertner.

Fig. 43. Indications of the 'Sterilization Law' of January 1934 in Nazi Germany, approved by the Chancellor of the Reich, Adolf Hitler.

At pseudo processes of the 'Erbgesundheitgerichten' the indication for sterilization and/or abortion was directed and as a consequence about 400.000 persons were made infertile during the Nazi regime. At German scientific otology society meetings at that time, compulsory sterilization or abortion often were serious topics of discussion. For example Wittmaack from Hamburg and Kahler from Freiburg were against this type of treatment of hereditary deafness, while Schwartz from Frankfurt and Mayer from Vienna were protagonists of compulsory sterilization as the only solution within the eugenic ideology.

In 1938, Prof. Nager from Zürich warned against inaccurate declarations in cases of otosclerosis for compulsory sterilization or abortion. He described a case in which a presumably otosclerosic pregnant patient was treated by Röntgen radiation of the gravis uterus according to the method advised in Laughlin's book *Eugenical sterilization in the United States*'. This abortion procedure had preference because it was believed that it resulted in a 'normal' end of the pregnancy. Unfortunately in Nager's case, the patient developed a lethal sepsis. Autopsy was performed on the temporal bone and revealed no sign of any histological otosclerosis.

Nager on the other hand, supported the ideas of Bell about hearing impaired patients avoiding marriages and offspring.

Greifenstein from München published papers in 1939 about abortion and sterilization in otosclerosis cases. These papers could be considered as guidelines for the German Reichsgutachterstelle to legalize in more detail these treatments for the eugenic reason of terminating the genetic disease otosclerosis. According to these guidelines, forty-three pregnant otosclerostic women had an abortion and twenty three were sterilized in 1939. The total number of pregnant otosclerotic woman who were treated by sterilization and/or abortion during the Nazi regime will never be known, but from the few data available it must have been at least hundreds to perhaps even over a thousand of cases. In 1938 in Los Angeles, Guggenheim pointed on the primary importance of avoidance of propagation in cases of otosclerosis, especially for the otosclerotic women, because of two reasons: the offspring could inherit the malady, and the mother could suffer from marked and rapid deterioration of her hearing as a result of the pregnancy. Guggenheim established a deafness prevention center.

According to Barton from Boston, abortion as treatment of pregnant women with severe otosclerosis to stop the hearing loss was not an infrequent procedure in the USA in the 1940s. In 1945, he described cases in which improvement of perceptive otosclerotic hearing was achieved after so-called therapeutic abortion.

In 1951, Pearson wrote a review in which he concluded that because otosclerosis and pregnancy often go together, termination of the pregnancy and sometimes sterilization might be considered as treatment in progressive cases of otosclerosis in pregnancy.

After the good results of the surgical treatment by stapes mobilization and later stapedectomy the role of otosclerosis in pregnancy became less important. In 1954, Walsh already found that there is no evidence of a relationship between pregnancy, hearing loss and otosclerosis. Precechtel (1967) on the other hand, found that pregnancy can aggravate the symptoms of otosclerosis. Hall *et al.* (1974) demonstrated that only 8% of the otosclerotic patients had an aggravation of hearing problems during their pregnancy. Later, in a retrospective study of 479 women with deafness from otosclerosis, Gristwood and Venables (1983) demonstrated that pregnancy does involve a risk of aggravating deafness in clinical otosclerosis. They reported a subjective deterioration in female patients with bilateral pregnancy-related otosclerosis that varied from about 33% after one pregnancy to about 63% after six pregnancies. In pregnant women with unilateral otosclerosis, deterioration of hearing was much less observed. There was no strong evidence that pregnancies cause any alteration to the actual footplate pathology of female patients. The introduction of the oral contraceptive pill did not influence the otosclerostic process, as demonstrated by Podoshin *et al.* (1974). Recently, Lippy *et al.* (2005) found no adverse effect on hearing in women with otosclerosis who had children compared with otosclerotic women without children. This age-adjusted study of 94 otosclerotic women revealed no negative effect caused by pregnancy on any outcome measurements like hearing levels. Also he demonstrated that there is no evidence of deterioration of hearing in otosclerotic women due to pregnancy. The role of pregnancy in the otosclerostic process seems to be rather small and any treatment of the past must be considered useless.

Chapter four

Surgical treatment of otosclerosis

1. Alternative surgical approach for otosclerosis

1.1. Wittmaack theory and treatment of otosclerosis

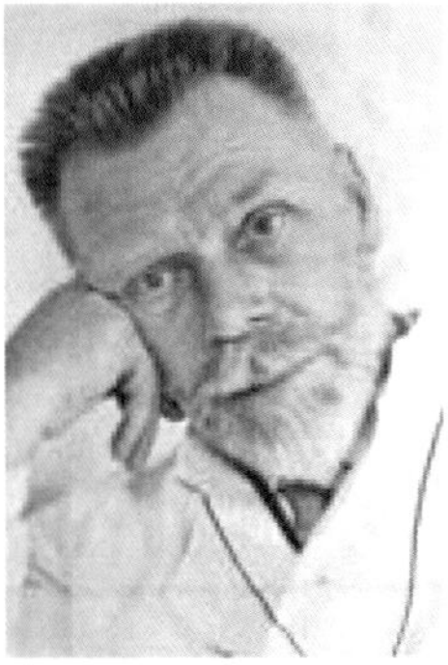

Fig. 44. Karl Wittmaack.

Karl Wittmaack (1876-1972; Fig. 44) in Jena and later Hamburg (Germany) performed many studies on the ethiology and the treatment of otosclerosis. He collected a huge number of temporal bones with all kinds of ear diseases. In a series of 1721 there were 90 temporal bones with otosclerosis.

In these bones, Wittmaack observed that the otosclerotic process started with a marked venous stasis within a selected area of the bony capsule of the inner ear. Already in 1870, Schwartze described the increased vascularity of the cochlear promontary during the active stage of otosclerosis, later known as Schwartze's sign. An otosclerotic zone was found around the enlarged vessels within which the bony substance was absorbed and its place was taken by tissue moderately rich in cells. Furthermore, Wittmaack and his group performed animal experiments to study the pathogenesis of otosclerosis. From the results of anatomical studies in chicken, Wittmaack concluded that venous stasis produced a retrograde blood transfer towards the labyrinth resulting in histological paterns that resemble otosclerosis found in human temporal bones.

Wittmaack was so convinced that his 'Stauungstheorie' on the pathogenesis of otosclerosis (Fig. 45) was the right one that he ended his final study on the subject with the following statements:

- Which other explanation (fundamental research) for otosclerosis is more able to combine the formal and causal genesis of otosclerosis than our theory?
- Which other explanation (fundamental research) is more able to present a full picture of the otosclerotic process from beginning to end than ours?

- Which other explanation (fundamental research) is more able to explain the morphological findings in combination with the clinical expression of the disease than our study?
- Last but not least. Which other series of studies resulted in so much well-documented clinical and experimental data as ours?

Fig. 45. Wittmaacks 'Stauungstheorie' for the pathogenesis of otosclerosis.

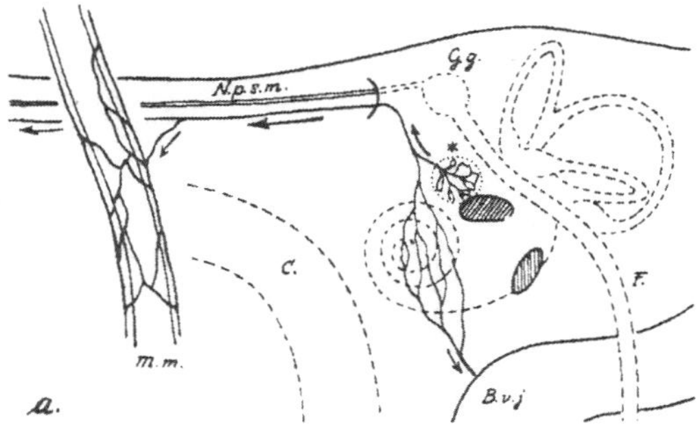

Abb. 9 *a*.

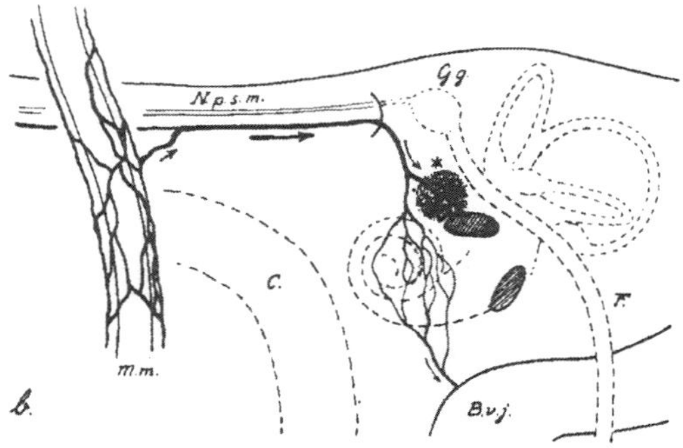

Abb. 9 *b*.

B. v. j. = Bulbus venae jugularis, *C* = Arteria carotis, *F* = Nervus facialis, *G. g.* = Ganglion geniculi, *m. m.* = Arteria meningea media, *N. p. s. m.* = Nervus petrosus superficialis major.

Abb. 9 *a*. Schematische Darstellung des *normalen* Venenstromes vom typischen Prädilektionsbezirk (*) zum Plexus der Arteria meningea media.

Abb. 9 *b*. ‚Schematische Darstellung des *pathologischen* rückläufigen Venenstromes vom Plexus der Arteria meningea media zum Otoskleroseherd an typischer Prädilektionsstelle (*).

1.2. Raising of the dura mater as treatment for otosclerosis

On the basis of these findings Wittmaack, Heyninx and Rollin developed an alternative surgical approach to attack the problem of the venous stasis near the anterior area next to the footplate of the stapes in cases of otosclerosis. The Wittmaack-Heyninx-Rollin method was devised by Wittmaack in 1918, and performed on cadavers by Heyninx in 1925. It had been carried out on patients since 1932, by Wittmaack and Rollin at Hamburg. The surgical procedure was also called 'soulèvement de la dure-mère supra-tympanique' (raising of the supra-tympanic dura mater). Its technique is endocranial, and consists in separating the dura mater from the antero-superior surface of the petrous bone, and thus lacerating the blood vessels. As a consequence there is a decrease of perilabyrinthine circulation and blood stagnation, which is generally considered to be the first anatomical lesion of the otosclerotic disease. This procedure had no direct effect on the actual lesions; its purpose was to stop the progress of deafness. The results of 20 procedures were demonstrated by Rollin in 1933 and showed that tinnitus was reduced, but that the outcome on the prevention of further deafness was doubtful. Rollin describes his results in a later publication as 70 to 80% positive. In the same publication, Rollin compares the Wittmaack operation with fenestration surgery and concludes that the Wittmaack operation does not damage the hearing and prevents further perceptive hearing loss, and that the fenestration approach is indicated when the Wittmaack operation is not applicable anymore. Von Nassuphis from Hamburg reported in 1951 the results of a 15 years follow-up of patients treated with the raising of the dura in cases of otosclerosis. Of circa 500 cases operated with this method he could only analyse 214 cases because of the loss of data due to the second world war. The results of this follow-up study showed that in 48,6 % of the cases the progression of the otosclerostic process could be stopped. Von Nassuphis concluded that the "Duralüftung" still had a place in the surgical treatment of otosclerosis notwithstanding the worldwide success of the fenestration techniques as introdued by Sourdille and Lempert in the 30's.

In 1950, the neurosurgeon Bordes-Valls from Valencia in Spain introduced a neurosurgical approach to fenestrate the semicircular canal after having seen five fenestration operations for otosclerosis. Through a temporal craniotomy, the dura was elevated until the arcuate eminence became visible. The tegmen tympani was then perforated and through the hole in the tegmen a window was made in the anterior portion of the lateral semicircular canal (Figs. 46 & 47). One case was reported by the author. After this initial paper, no results of this approach have been documented any more.

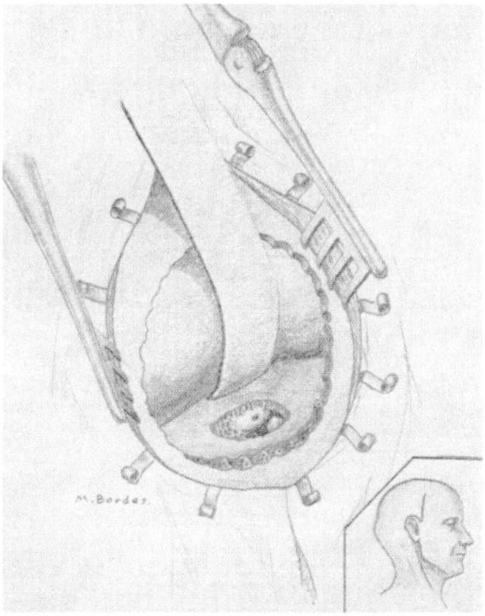

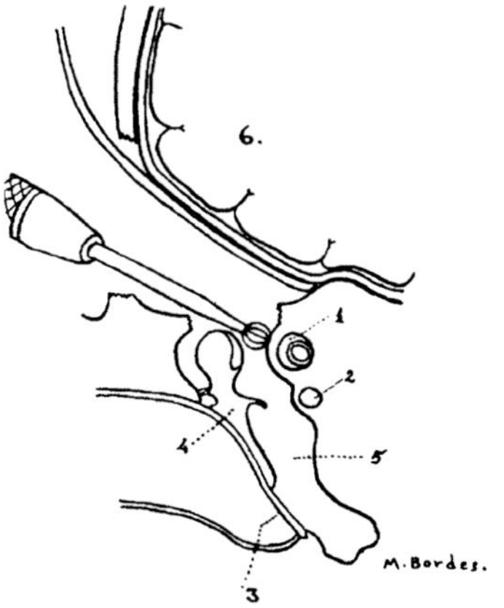

Fig. 2.—Schematic representation of the production of the fenestra. *1,* External semicircular canal; *2,* facial nerve; *3,* tympanic membrane; *4,* malleus; *5,* middle ear; *6,* brain.

Fig. 46 (left). Original drawing of the neurosurgical approach to fenestrate the semicircular canal by Bordes-Valls

Fig. 47 (right). Schematical drawing of the neurosurgical approach of Bordes-Valls

In 1961, William House and neurosurgeon Theodore Kurze performed 14 cadaveric dissections to refine the middle-fossa approach. This approach was already described by Panse and Parry in 1904 to treat tinnitus and vertigo by division of the vestibulocochlear nerve. After having gained experience in the experimental stage, the middle-fossa approach was performed with the aid of an operating microscope for decompression of the internal auditory canal in the management of cases with otosclerosis. This neurosurgical treatment for otosclerosis was unsuccessful and was abandoned. In 1963, House perfected the middle-cranial-fossa approach for acoustic neuromas removal. This approach proved to be very successful in the treatment of these tumours in the internal auditory meatus.

2. Fenestration of the labyrinth

2.1. The development of the fenestration surgery as treatment for otosclerosis

In 1910 more than a decennium after Passow, Floderus and Ballance experimented with a fistula in the labyrinth for the treatment of otosclerosis Róbert Bárány (1876-1936; Fig. 48) from Vienna in Austria again suggested surgery in cases of otosclerosis. A fenestra fistula in the posterior semicircular canal after a large mastoidectomy was his surgical approach. He obtained good results and the success lasted longer than just a few weeks. However, after a fatal complication of the fenestra surgery for otosclerosis in his tenth patient, Bárány stopped with that approach for the treatment of otosclerosis.

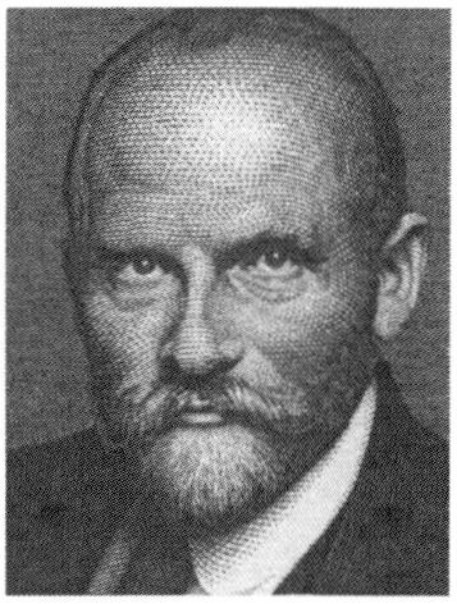

Fig. 48. Róbert Bárány.

At an international congress of medicine in London in 1913, Jenkins reported two operations; one a posterior opening through a simple incision with a trephining of the horizontal canal with a electric drill, and another in which an opening was made in the horizontal canal and a plastic flap was cut from the posterior meatal wall and spread on the floor of the cavity to cover the fenestration. Jenkins was the first to make such an opening which he called 'fenestration' in the external or lateral semicircular canal, but sadly enough, hearing improvement did not last long. Bárány and Jenkins discussed the problem of possible ossification of the fenestra at the same congress in London. During the first world war, Bárány was a surgeon in the Austrian army. He was captured by the Russians and was held in a camp as prisoner of war when the Nobel Prize was awarded to him in 1914. After his release in 1916 he went to Sweden, where he met Holmgren in Stockholm.

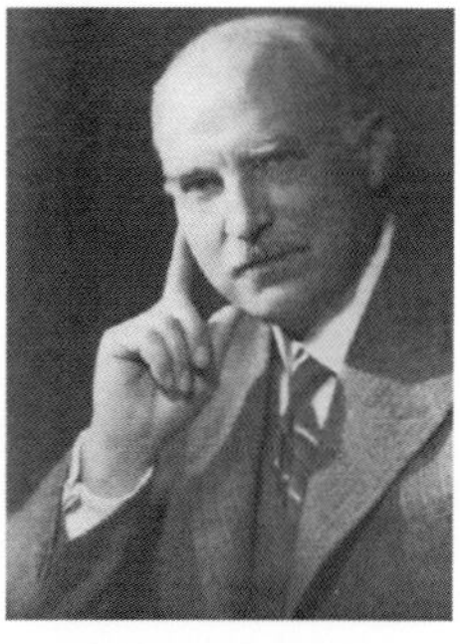

Fig. 49. Gunnar Holmgren.

Bárány and Holmgren (1875-1954; Fig. 49) both believed that decompression of the perilymphatic space was the solution for the cure of otosclerosis. Holmgren suggested to make an opening in

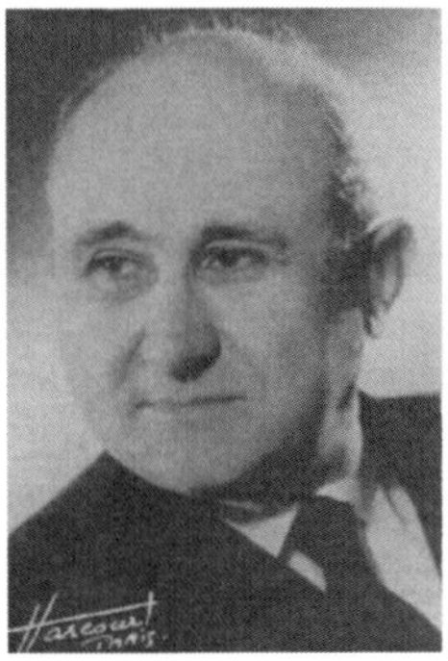

Fig. 50. Maurice Sourdille.

the superior semi-circular canal, which could be covered by the dura, hoping to delay or prevent bone closure.

The French otologist Maurice Sourdille (1885-1961; Fig. 50) from Nantes visited Bárány and Holmgren in October 1924 in Sweden and he was impressed by their extremely delicate surgical approach to create fenestra in the inner ear to treat otosclerosis. Back in France, Sourdille combined this surgical technique with some of his own elements and called it 'tympanolabyrinthopexy'. According to Sourdille, the surgery should be performed in total aseptic conditions and the best results would be obtained in two or even three stages. Sourdille presented his surgical approach and first results on 16 & 17 December in 1929 at the Société d'Otologie des Hopitaux in Paris. In September 1930 his paper on the subject was published (Fig. 51).

The Journal of
Laryngology and Otology
(Founded in 1887 by MORELL MACKENZIE *and* NORRIS WOLFENDEN)
September 1930

ON THE SURGICAL TREATMENT OF OTOSCLEROSIS.

By MAURICE SOURDILLE, Nantes.
(Assistant Professor of Surgery at the School of Medicine, Nantes.)

Fig. 51. The international paper by Sourdille presenting his first results of the fenestration.

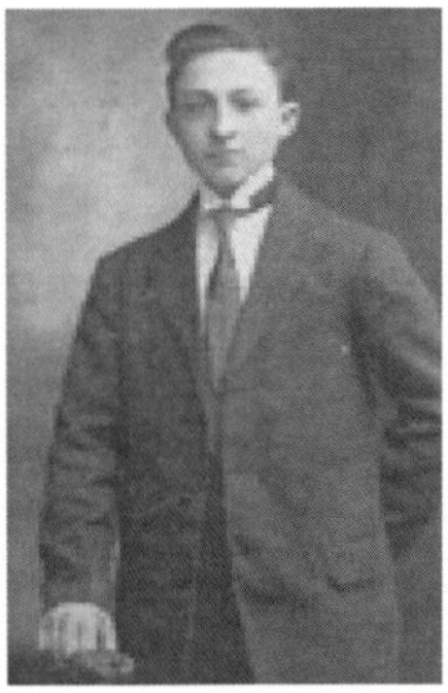

Fig. 52. Young Julius Lempert.

In 1937, Sourdille was invited to the USA by Fowler to present a lecture (October 6) and to perform the surgery at the New York Academy of Medicine.

At that meeting Sourdille met the young otolaryngologist Lempert (1890-1968; Fig. 52). Lempert was impressed by the work of Sourdille and suggested the one-stage endaural approach which he had introduced for chronic infected mastoid surgery. Lempert introduced the one-stage endaural approach for the fenestration of the lateral semi-circular canal in 1938. In that same year, G.E. Shambaugh jr. was a guest in the operation theatre where Lempert was performing a one-stage fenestration in local aneasthesia. The patient could hear better after the horizontal canal was opened and Shambaugh was convinced of this treatment for otosclerosis. This fenestration operation of the horizontal semi-circular canal was the surgical treatment of choice in cases of otosclerosis for almost two decades.

2.2. Fenestration operation

The approach towards the labyrinth for the fenestration of the inner ear was:

- Retroauricular (Sourdille), or
- Endaural (Lempert), or
- Preauricular (Popper).

2.2.1. Fenestration according to Maurice Sourdille

Jenkins, Bárány and Holmgren showed that opening of the labyrinth could result in better hearing in cases of otosclerosis. Encouraged by the experiences of these pioneers in fenestration surgery, Sourdille started to work on an improved procedure. He came up with a technique which requires a double-staged operation. The first stage was to explore the middle ear and to isolate it. It was an attico-tympanotomy canal-wall-down combined with an internal plastic with a tympanic hinge. The second operation opens the canalis semicircularis externus aseptically and occludes this fenestration by a thin epidermic membrane. Both staged operations were performed under local anaesthesia and with strong adrenalisation.

A mastoid trepanation was performed with very careful elevation of the soft parts of the external auditory canal from the bone, followed by mobilization of the tympanic membrane, only in the upper half of its circumference, with the cutaneous lining of the external auditory canal. The next step was a resection of the osseous bridge of the external wall of the attic and of the tympanic ring, corresponding to the portion of the tympanic membrane to be mobilised. A large view of the attic, the tympanic cavity and the ossicles was thus created. Sourdille called this a simple attico-tympanotomy; it permits the exploration of the ossicles (Fig. 53).

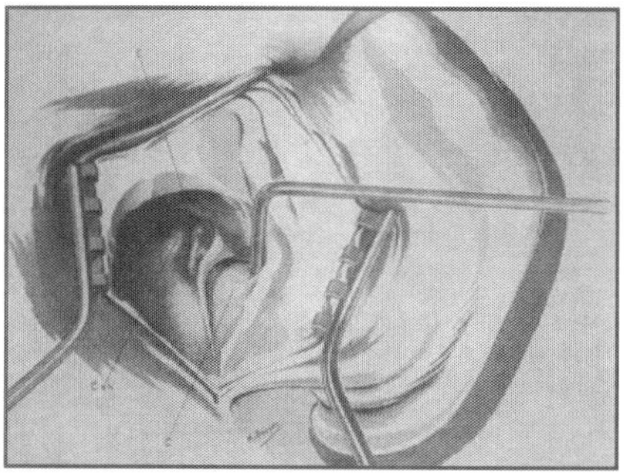

Fig. 53. Sourdille's first-stage operation for fenestration.

The incus was then removed with or without resection of the caput mallei to obtain a good view on the bony horizontal semicircular canal (Fig. 54). Now a skin flap with tympanic hinge was obtained from the postero-superior wall of the membranous canal and was lowered inwardly against the internal wall of the attic. By its adherence to this wall, the tympanic cavity was hermetically closed and separated from the mastoid region (Fig. 55).

This ended the first stage of Sourdille's fenestration. The postoperative treatment consists of dressings, continued until the epidermisation of the mastoid cavity.

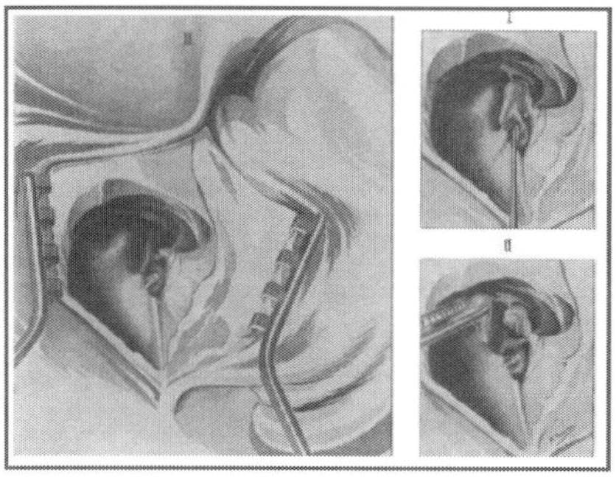

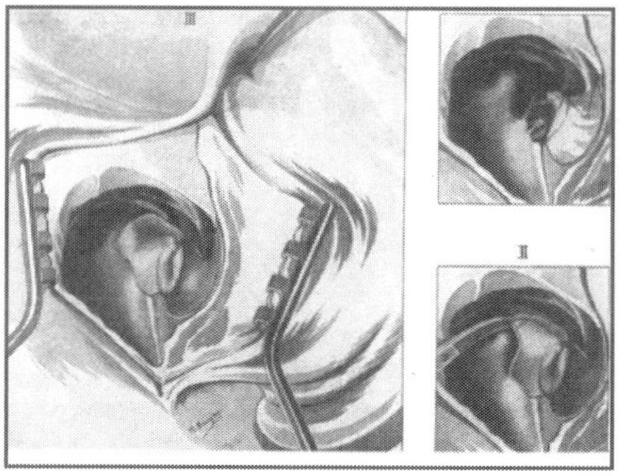

Fig. 54 (left). Removal of the incus after removal of the bony external canal wall.

Fig. 55 (right). Preparing the tympanomeatal flap to cover the horozontal canal.

The second stage, consisting of a trepanation of the prominence of the external semicircular canal, was performed a few months later, when the cicatricial lining of the mastoid cavity was sufficiently thin and transparent. The retro-auricular wound was reopened with cutting out of the cicatricial flap that was used to cover the region of the semicircular canal. The tympanic cavity should not be opened yet (Fig. 56).

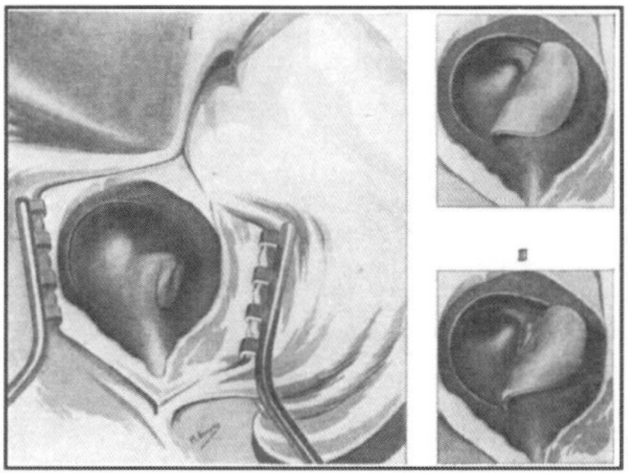

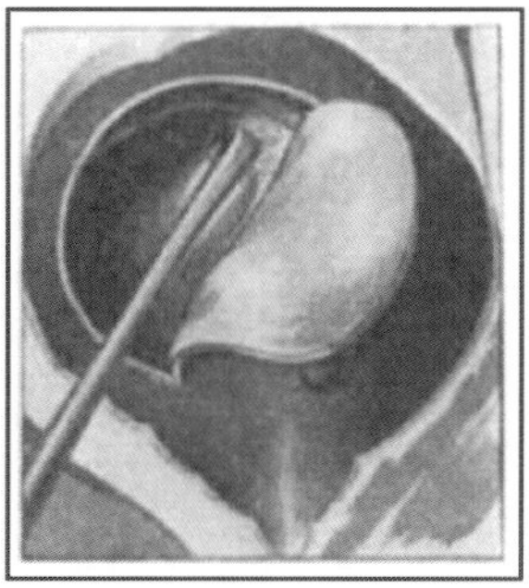

Fig. 56 (left). Second stage of the fenestration technique of sourdille : re-opening of the mastoid cavity

Fig. 57 (right). Preparation of the fenestration by rubbing.

The next step was trepanation of the prominence of the external semicircular canal by rubbing of that area with special rubbers (Fig. 57). Then the epidermic flap was placed on the orifice of labyrinthine fenestration, closing it off to prevent infection of the internal ear. This flap was maintained by applying paraffined gauze meshes up to the moment of full cicatrisation of the entire mastoid cavity (Fig. 58).

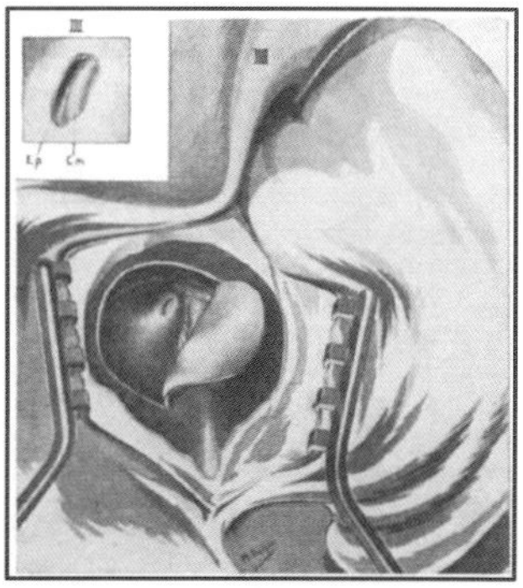

Fig. 58. End of the second stage by placing the flap upon the fenestration.

Sourdille defended the two stage approach for the sake of caution. As he stated in 1930 the surgical treatment of otosclerosis was only at the very beginning and great caution must necessarily be exercised. Inflammatory reaction which may follow the opening of the tympanic cavity can occur and with an open labyrinth immediately at the same procedure runs the great risk of infection of the labyrinth so that all eventual success would be compromised. Further more the preparation of the plastic epidermic strip which must re-cover the labyrinthine trepanation could be difficult or insufficient in some cases so that it will be worthy to have a pause between the creation of the attico-tympanotomy cavity and the fenestration of the labyrinth. Sourdille stated that it was necessary to open the labyrinth by slow and progressive rubbing of the bone with special rubbers. He had invented special rubber which he demonstrated at the meeting the Societe de Laryngologie des Hopitaux de Paris 17th December 1929. He was against the perforation of the labyrinth with a burr. Although Sourdille advocated the second staged approach for the fenestration operation for otosclerosis he also experienced a newer technique, requiring only a single operation. His experience with this one stage fenestration was discussed at the Franco-Belgian Meeting on Otology in Brussels on 4th June in 1930.

2.2.2. Fenestration according to Julius Lempert

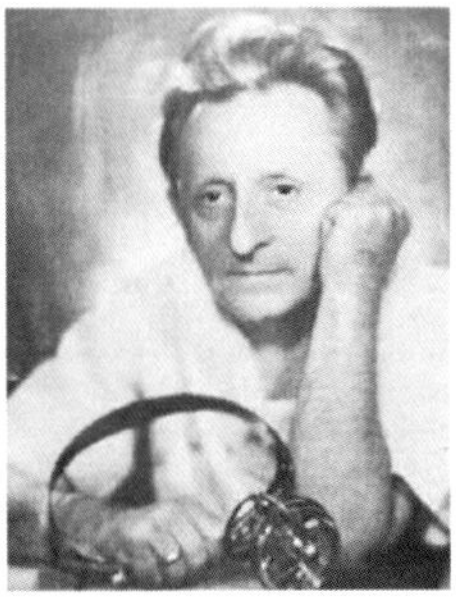

Fig. 59. Julius Lempert.

Julius Lempert (1890-1968; Fig. 59) who attended Sourdille's lecture and demonstration in New York, was impressed by what he heard and saw. He invited Sourdille for dinner and asked him all about the details of the so-called tympanolabyrinthopexy procedure for otosclerosis surgery. After this meeting, Lempert started to develop the one-stage endaural approach for the fenestration of the lateral semi-circular canal.

His procedure was a combination of the endaural approach introduced by Hans Heermann (1930) and Sourdille's method (1929) (Fig. 60). A new element was the introduction of the dental surgical burr to open the mastoid and to expose the horizontal semicircular canal. The creation of the fenestra was done with a plug finishing burr instead of the little scraper with rubber to make the opening in the horizontal canal that Sourdille used. To close the fenestra, Lempert used the same method as Sourdille. At that time no otologist in the U.S.A was performing any type of surgery for restoring the hearing in cases of otosclerosis. Lempert was a brilliant ear surgeon and he was very successful

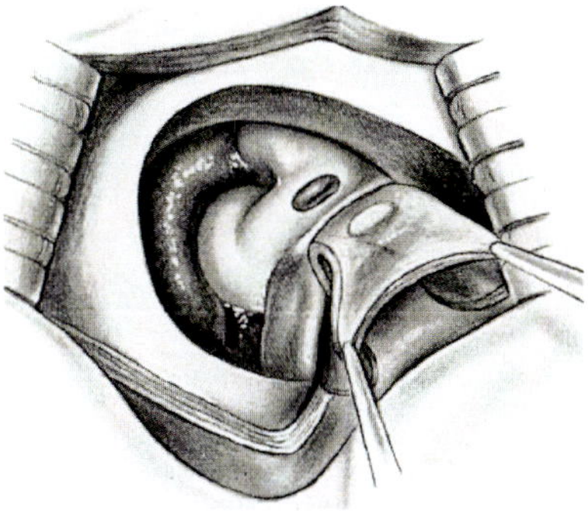

Fig. 60. Lempert's one-stage approach for the fenestration of the horizontal canal.

with his modified one-stage fenestration approach. In 1938, he reported his first 23 cases of hearing restoration with this new surgical technique, but he scarcely refer to or cite the work of Sourdille. On the other hand, Sourdille did not mention the work of Lempert in his monography from 1955 entitled *Tendances évolutive de la fénestration*. Soon after Lempert's first success, prominent American otologists came to observe Lempert's surgery. One of them was George Shambaugh, Jr. of Chicago, who was greatly impressed by the operation and Lempert's surgical skill. Shambaugh immediately introduced Lempert's fenestration surgery in his clinic.

Lempert initiated a temporal bone course twice a year for ear surgeons who were interested in his technique, promoting his surgical approach for the treatment of otosclerosis.

A clinical picture of the middle ear and mastoid cavity after a fenestration is shown in Figure 61.

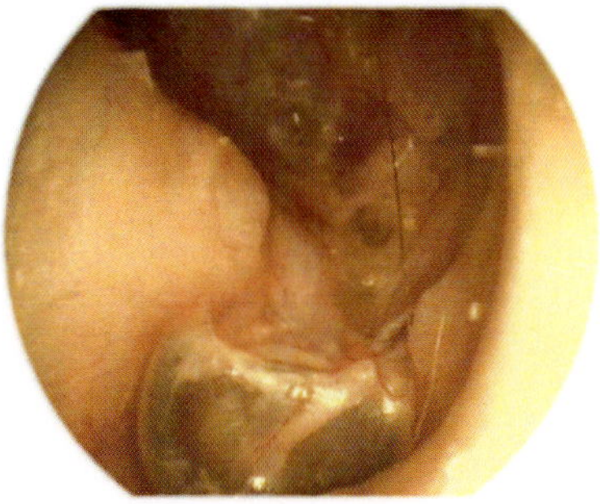

Fig. 61. A clinical picture of a fenestration of the right ear.

2.2.3. Fenestration according to Oswald Otto Popper

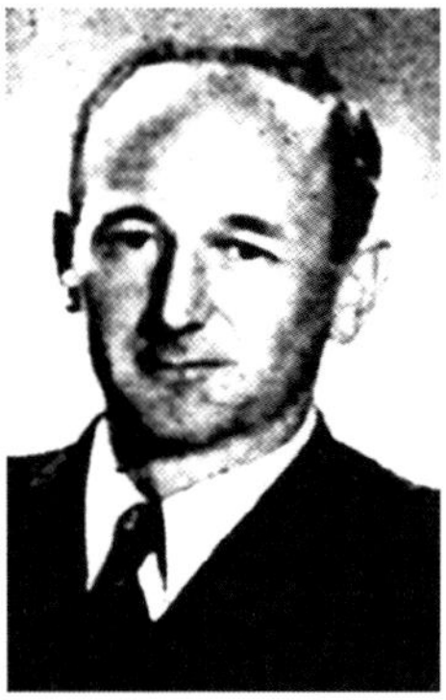

Fig. 62. Otto Popper.

Stimulated by Lempert's surgical fenestration technique for otosclerosis Oswald Popper (1899-1957; Fig. 62) from Johannesburg, South Africa conceived a different easier gateway to the labyrinth. In 1946, he introduced an alternative endaural approach for the fenestration of the labyrinth.

In those days, the treatment of otosclerosis consisted of the creating of a fenestrum and means of a flap with minimal tissue trauma. Popper invented the transtympanic route without opening the mastoid and without creating a radical cavity. Popper disagreed with Lempert about where the mastoid had to be opened and commented on the angle to perform the fenestration in Lempert's approach. He described a seven-steps preaural transtympanic approach without opening the mastoid (Fig. 63 a-l).

The procedure started with a preaural skin incision (1½ cm) just before the tragus to ensure a minimal scar (Fig. 63a). The skin was then lifted off the cartilage of the tragus; blunt dissection was performed to the bone of the cranial part of the external ear canal. The skin was then elevated from the canal wall and a second incision in the canal skin was made to open the external ear canal. Then a flap was created from the skin of the upper wall of the auditory canal (Fig. 63 b & c). This meatal-skin flap stayed attached to the malleus long process and the tympano membrane and elevated from the posterial bony ear canal. The elevated skin flap was folded over the malleus in the ear canal (Fig. 63 d & e). With diamond burrs the attic wall above the incus was removed, followed by removal of the incus to expose the dome of the vestibule (Fig. 63 f & g). With the burr, a fenestration of the dome of the vestibule was then performed (Fig. 63 h-j). The eardrum was placed back in position, the superior meatal ear canal skin flap was pushed inside to cover the fistula of the fenestration. Vaseline gauze strips were placed to pack the meatus and the preaual incision was closed (Fig. 63 k & l).

Fig. 63 (a - l). The Popper approach for the fenestration of the labyrinth without opening the mastoid.

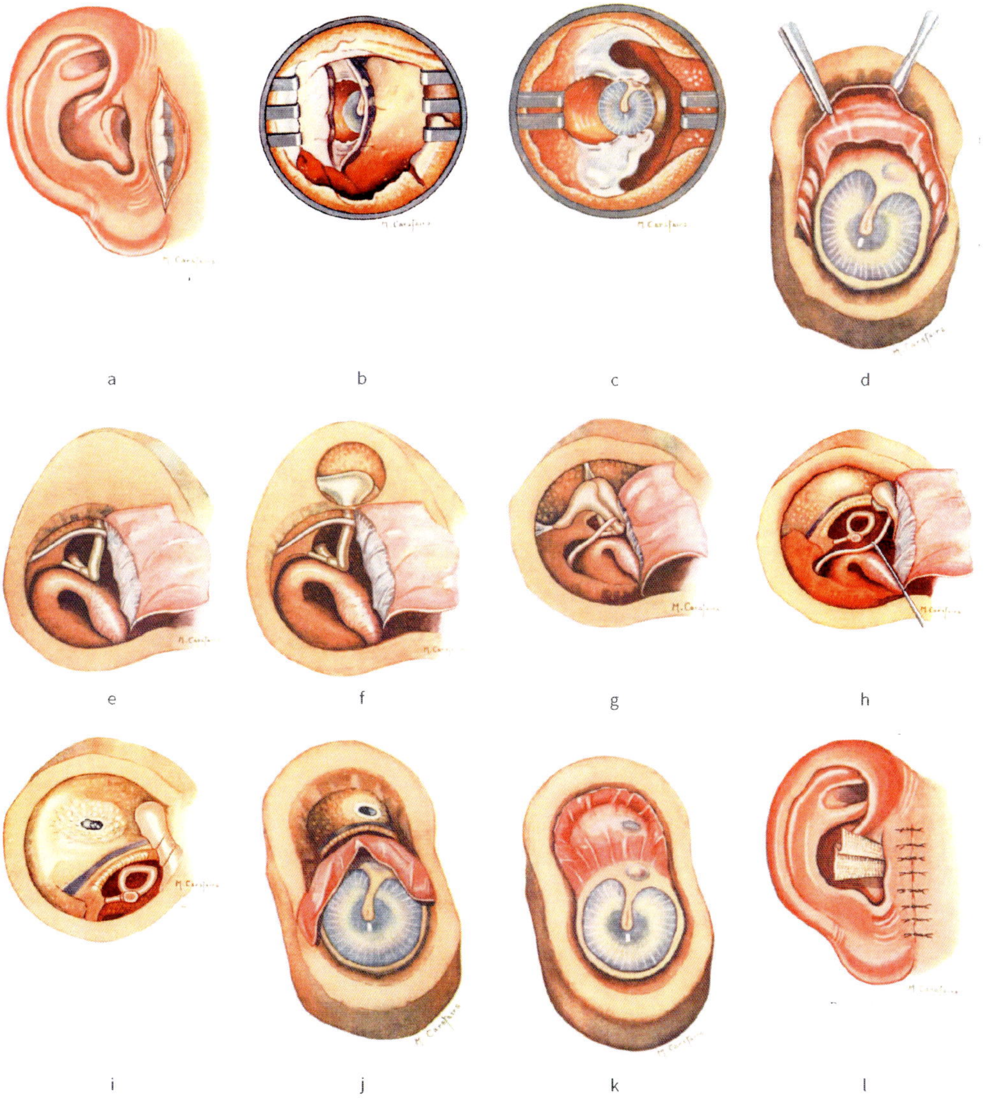

The advantages of this approach were:

- The tympano-meatal flap could be detached easily and quickly, without time being wasted on thinning and breaking down the posterior bony meatal wall;
- The tympanic membrane was only detached to a small extent and did not have to be stretched;
- A 'square-on' view of the site of fenestration in the vestibular dome;
- The facial canal was clearly seen;
- The mastoid was kept intact;
- There was no need to remove the malleus head;
- There was considerably less operative trauma to middle ear.

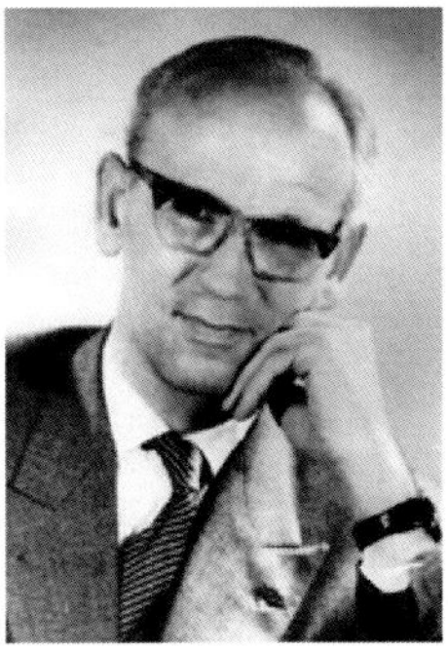

Fig. 64. Leonard Jongkees.

The results of the Popper transtympanic fenestration approach varied between 50% (Poulsen) to 75,5% (Meurman) in hearing improvement. In 1950, Leonard Jongkees (1912-2002; Fig. 64) from Amsterdam, after having performed this procedure in 25 cases, pointed out some disadvantages of the technique. The space obtained by the preaural approach is very limited, which makes visualisation difficult and instrumentation a very delicate affair. The square-on view of the site of fenestration in the vestibular dome is good for orientation, but makes the drilling of the fenestra a difficult procedure. Since the fenestra was made at the deepest point of the cavity, it was almost impossible to prevent the entrance of blood or bone dust into the labyrinth in 100% of cases. The facial nerve stands out clearly, thus presenting the advantage of clear visibility, but also requiring extreme surgical skills. Even the slightest wrong move (easily made in this extremely small space) could cause injury to the facial nerve.

Jongkees also stated that in some selected cases of early cholesteatoma or polyposis of the attic, the Popper approach seemed very promising. In 1956, Bauer documented serious side effects of the preaural transtympanic Popper approach. In some cases a post-operative stenosis of the external ear canal was the result, a complication that required a reoperation consisting of a conservative radical cavity.

2.2.4. The problem of the osteogenetic closure of the newly created fenestra in the fenestration surgery for otosclerosis

Bárány and Jenkins, the pioneers of the fenestration of the labyrinth already discussed the problem of possible ossification of the fenestra on a congress in London in 1913. Holmgren and Sourdille observed that short after a fenestration (Fig. 65), the improvement in hearing diminished to the pre-operative status. Lempert found the same result and he noticed in his follow up that after fenestration surgery, osteogenetic closure of the newly-created fenestra occurred (Fig. 66).

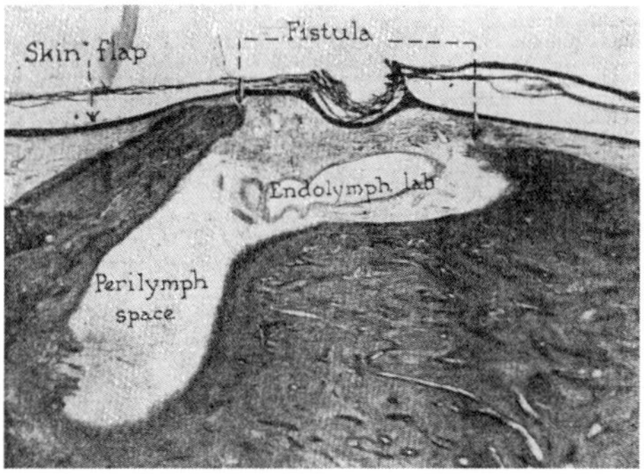

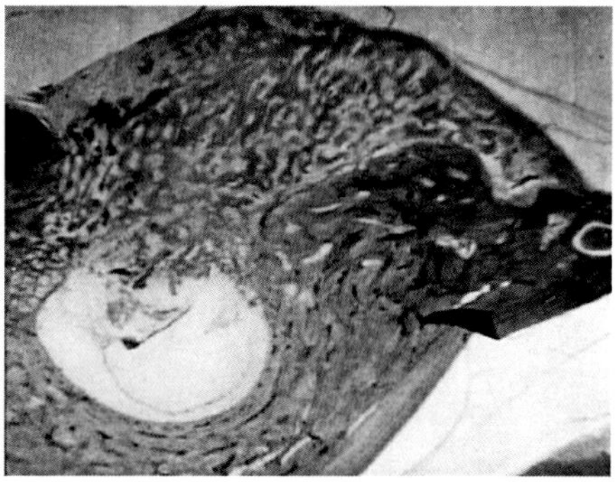

Fig. 65 (left). Histology of an open fenestra of the horizontal canal.

Fig. 66 (right). Histology of an osteogenetic closure of the created fenestra.

This closure was the reason that permanent maintenance of the early hearing improvement obtained by fenestration surgery failed in many cases. In an animal study on Rhesus monkeys, Lempert burnished the fenestra rim with different metals and it seemed that gold and lead prevented the osteogenesis. To understand this natural repair within the bony labyrinthine capsule after fenestration, Lempert studied cases in which osteogenetically closed post-operative labyrinthine fenestras had occurred. He concluded that when bone dust was left in the region of the fenestra, closure occurs and that this process started in the innermost endosteal bony layer of the fenestra. As a result of these studies, a gold burnishing burr was advocated to prepare the fenestration and to apply lead on the edges of the fenestra. Also important was the fact that during the surgery all bone dust must be meticulously removed to prevent closure in the fenestra post-operatively. After analysis of his observations during revisions of bony closed fenestras, Lempert developed his fenestra nov-ovalis technique in 1941. He changed the fenestra site by moving it forward to the ampulla of the external semicircular canal and prepared a somewhat larger window closer to the labyrinth vestibule. Because he placed the fenestra in that region, osteogenetic closure of the fenestra was less likely. The results of the fenestration treatment improved but osteogenetic closure remained a problem. In 1945, Lempert introduced the mobile cartilage stopple to fight this problem (Fig. 67).

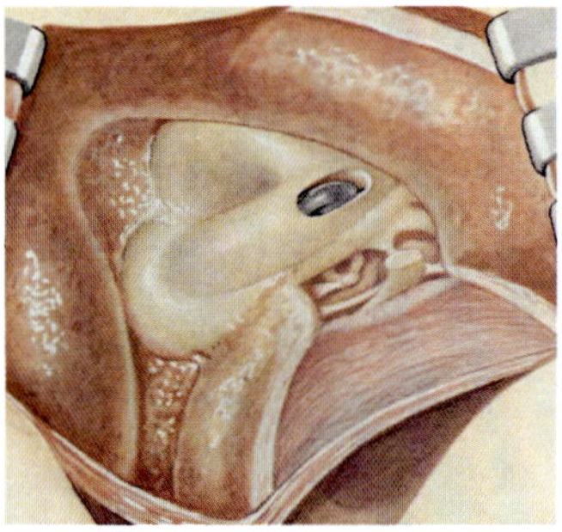

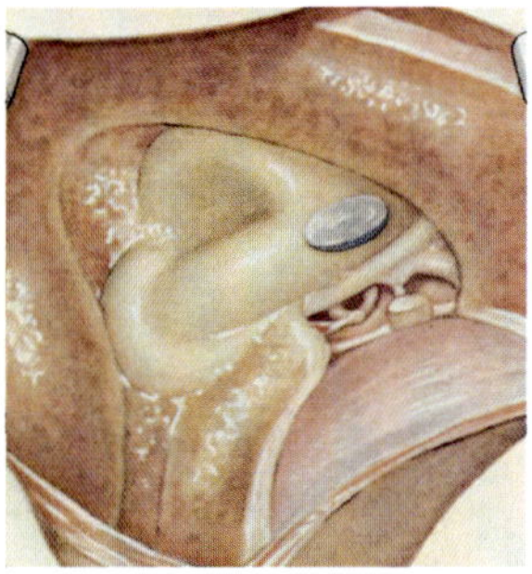

Fig. 67a & 67b. The creation of the 'stopple' invented by Lempert.

A small piece of cartilage was taken from the pinna and used as a cork to cover the fenestra. This introduction of an autogenous cartilage 'stopple' graft initially had some success. When Aubry (1946) used an acrylite stopple instead of a cartilaginous one, however, it did not entirely prevent closure of the fenestra and development of serous labyrinthitis.

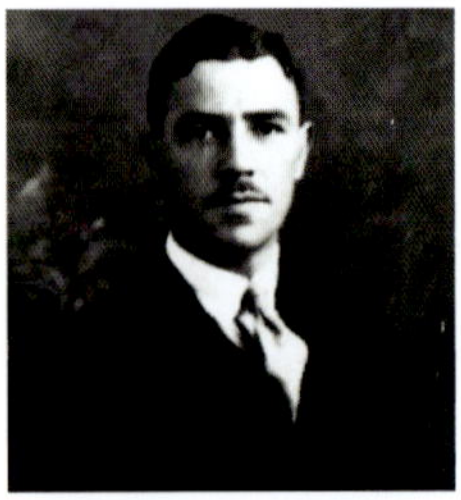

Fig. 68. Roland Garnett Passe.

In 1947, Garnett Passe (1904-1952; Fig. 68) applied cartilage stopples in 100 cases of fenestration surgery for otosclerosis (Table 5), but ceased using this method, as in 10-15% of these cases a revision had to be carried out because the cartilage stopple was found to be immobilized or even to have been extruded by fibrous tissues. He propagated a much larger fenestration as shown in Figure 69 to overcome this problem. Lempert admitted in 1951 that he had to abandon his own invention of the cartilage stopple for the same reasons as mentioned by Garnett Passe.

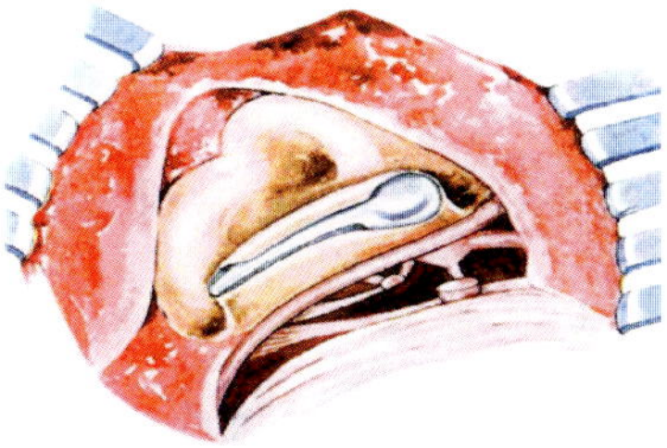

Fig. 69. The large fenestration as proposed by Garnett Passe in 1948.

Table 5. Results of the use of the cartilage stopple by Garnett Passe.

INTERIM RESULTS

Series	Total no. of cases	Hearing never improved	Hearing improved but improvement lost later	Hearing worse	Hearing improved and fully maintained
1936/39	36	5	28	1	2 of 8 years' duration
1945/46 with cochlear stopple	100	7	36	2	53 of 1-2 years' duration
1946/47 enchrondralized fistula	136	11	2	none	153 during last 12 months

Another method for preventing obliteration of the fenestra was the use of a Thiersch's graft to cover the new window with invagination in the fenestra. It was applied by Brunner (1948) and later Siirala (1952). In spite of all these efforts like different sites of the fenestra (Fig. 70) to prevent osteogenetic closure of the fenestra window, it continued to be unpredictable which of the created windows would close

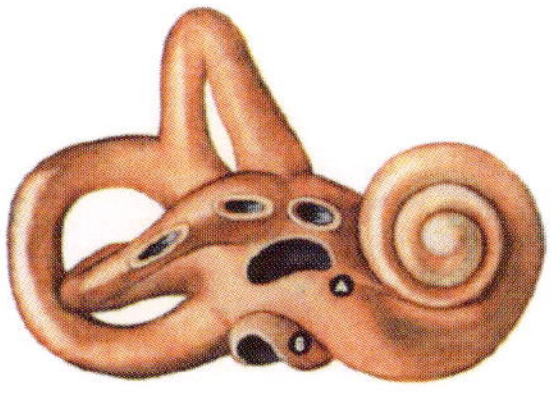

Fig. 70. Different positions of the fenestration.

and which would remain open. The nov-ovalis technique with intra-marginal invagination of the tympanomeatal flap in the window did diminish, but not completely prevent osteogenetic closure of the newly-created fenestra. Table 6. shows the different type of stopple's to prevent reossification of the fenestration used in revision surgery.

Table 6. Different materials applied to prevent reclosure of the fenestration.

Fenestration revision	Type of 'Stopple'
Aubry	Acrylite stopple
Scott-Brown	Plastic or tantalum stopple
Lempert	Cartilage stopple
Ombredanne	Skin graft
Moser	Buccal mucosa
Rosen	Chorda tympani
Garson	Eye conjuctiva

2.2.5. Results of the fenestration surgery

The first results of early fenestration surgery for otosclerosis were decribed by Sourdille in 1930. He published his second-stage procedure and presented the first results of six cases. Of these six patients, five were female. Post-operative follow up varied from six weeks to one year. The male patient lost his hearing during the follow-up period. In one case hearing improved, but the patient post-operatively suffered from intense tinnitus. It was noted that in all six cases low sounds were heard best. Generally, hearing was proportionately better for high sounds than for low sounds. Hearing improvement was not only a matter of intensity but, and more especially, also of clearness and distinction of hearing. This improvement in hearing for 'ordinary purposes' was observed by all the patients' friends and relations, except in one case.

Therefore, Sourdille concluded that his method proved that if the fenestra ovalis is blocked by the stapes, it is possible to restore hearing to a large extent by creating a labyrinthine fenestra in the curve of the horizontal canal. In Sourdille's opinion this was true, even if there were neuro-epithelial changes in the membranous labyrinth at the same time. In his comments he remarked that recovery of hearing appears to depend on the following factors:

- The degree of deafness before the operation;
- The decompression of the perilymph;
- The size of the artificial orifice.

Direct access to the labyrinth of sound waves by means of this orifice in the curve of the horizontal canal, and any obstacle intervening between the perilymph and the outer air diminishes hearing. In 1937, Sourdille presented the results of his surgical approach for otosclerosis until 1935. He had treated 109 patients and performed a total of 325 operations. He claimed a positive result in 74% of these cases. He divided his results in categories:

- Very good results, *i.e.*, an increase to ten times (or more) the previous hearing distance, achieved in 40% of the cases;
- Good results, *i.e.*, an increase to five to ten times the previous hearing distance, achieved in 14% of the cases;
- Mediocre results, *i.e.*, an increase to two to five times the previous hearing distance, achieved in 20% of the cases;
- No fatalities.

Sourdille made an important observation: the labyrinthine fistula closed due to the reconstitution of a rigid bony layer, rarely attaining the thickness of the primitive bony wall of the canal, and more often not exceeding a few tenths of a millimeter. In those cases a second operation was needed to extract the bony film, in order to see the hearing gained with the first operation return. Sometimes this gain in hearing was even considerably increased after the second operation. In many cases, Sourdille had to re-open the labyrinth even three times to obtain a lasting result. In 1937 he had 140 patients, on whom a total of 400 operations were performed. At that time Lempert had not yet performed any fenestration surgery. The large numbers of revisions needed by Sourdille may have been the reason for Lempert to start working on a one-stage procedure for surgical treatment of otosclerosis. In May 1938, Lempert presented his development and a description of a one-stage fenestration technique, which made this surgery practical for both patient and otologist. The results of his first 23 cases were excellent and he claimed a hearing improvement of 80%. George Shambaugh (1903-1999; Fig. 71), who had adopted the surgical approach of Lempert, stated in 1941 that out of 201 cases he operated, 182 showed an improvement of hearing lasting for over a year. In 33% of those cases the gain amounted to more than 30 decibels.

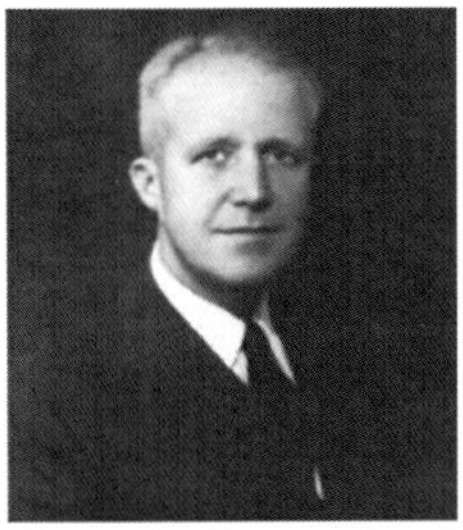

Fig. 71. George E. Shambaugh Jr.

In Great Britain, I. Simpson Hall (1946) decribed the results of his series of 118 fenestration operations using the approach of Lempert: making an opening at the far forward-end of the horizontal canal and placing cartilage to prevent closure of the fenestration. In 82 patients hearing improved, a success rate of approximately 69%. He discovered that in the group of patients of over 40 years of age the success rate was higher (80%). In his series, Simpson Hall had one case of facial paralysis, which recovered completely, and no cases of labyrinthitis. However, two fatalities occurred (resulting from acute cardiac arrest and from acute morphine poisoning).

In an overview of the results of fenestration surgery for otosclerosis, Holmgren (1948) made it clear that operative risks were relatively small. He stated that it was possible to achieve an immediate improvement of hearing. Nevertheless, in rare cases, it could also happen that hearing deteriorated or vanished altogether, and sometimes the facial nerve could be injured during the operation. In most of the cases, however, such an injury was transitory and was to be regarded as an extremely uncommon accident. Sometimes the operation wound could become infected, leading to a longer healing process and possibly other, more serious, complications. Dizziness was fairly common during the first post-operative weeks. In rare cases, this could be more pronounced and long-lasting. Achieved hearing improvement was far from permanent. In a large number of cases hearing regressed after a shorter or longer period, and then usually returned to the pre-operative condition. In such cases, hearing could sometimes be improved by performing a new operation. Normal hearing could never be achieved, but it could be improved to such a degree that the patient could carry on his work and associate with other people, practically undisturbed by his defect. Tinnitus in the ear usually would diminish after the operation, but could return when the hearing improvement regressed.

Different authors applied different criteria to analyze long-term results of surgery for otosclerosis based on fenestration of the labyrinth.

In 1951, Adin and Shambaugh documented a long-term study on the results of fenestration surgery (Fig. 72) in which partial loss of the regained hearing occurred in about one-fifth of the

Most Recent Hearing Result in
2,100 Consecutive Fenestration Operations

	Original Lempert Operation		Same with Cont. Irrig. and/or Micro.		Nov-ovalis with Irr. and Microscope		Cartilage Stopple Technic		Northwest. Improved Operation	
Date	1938-1940		1940		1940-1945		1944		1946-1949	
	No. of Cases	%	No. of Cases	%	No. of Cases	%	No. of Cases	%	No. of Cases	%
Hearing Worse	2	13.3	1	1.1	39	4.7	1	12.5	13	1.1
Hearing Unchanged	3	20	4	4.8	66	8.0			85	7.4
Improvement Lost	6	40	24	25.8	43	5.2			36	3.1
Total Not Improved	11	73.3	29	31.7	148	17.9	1	12.5	134	11.6
Gain Partly Lost	1	6.7	27	29.0	76	9.2	3	36.8	71	6.2
Gain Maintained +11 to +19 db	3	20	9	9.7	126	15.2	3	36.8	240	20.7
Gain Maintained +20 to 29 db.			13	13.9	252	30.4			455	39.4
Gain Maintained +30 to 60 db.			15	16.1	228	27.5	1	12.5	254	22.0
Total Improved	4	26.7	64	68.7	682	82.3	7	86.1	1,020	88.3
At 30 db. Practical Level	0		22	23.9	257	30.3	1	12.5	456	39.5

Fig. 72. Long-term results of 2100 fenestrations for otosclerosis by Shambaugh *et al.*

cases followed for five to ten years after fenestration. This loss was believed to be the result of either osteogenic narrowing of the fenestra, post-operative hydrops, or cochlear nerve degeneration, while in some cases no probable cause could be determined. In the majority of cases (70%) followed up for five to ten years, the level of hearing measured at the one-year post-operative test was maintained without noticeable change.

Rüedi *et al.* (1951) distinguished three groups of otosclerotic patients according to their suitability for fenestration operation, a distinction that could be made pre-operatively. The first group of cases was considered ideal for this type of operation. This group would have hearing loss by air of 35-45 dB for speech frequencies, while the bone conduction audiogram within the same range would look approximately normal. Accordingly, the Rinne test with the 1,024 Hz fork should be negative. The second group would have hearing loss by air of 40-60 dB for speech frequencies. The bone conduction would be below normal, but up to 2,000 Hz it would attain a level still clearly higher than -30 dB. The Rinne test should again be negative. The third group contained what were considered borderline cases. The audiogram would show a profound hearing impairment of 60-80 dB for speech frequencies. The bone conduction audiogram would show a clear descent within the range of 2,000 Hz or even below and would be below the critical level of -30 dB. The Rinne test should still be negative. Considering the great loss of air conduction in the so-called borderline cases with pronounced hearing impairment of the inner ear, fenestration could only produce useful results in a certain number of patients.

According to these criteria, hearing rehabilitation sufficient for practical purposes was found in 94.5% of ideal and suitable cases in a follow up after two years. Results in the borderline group were less favorable: only 50% were successfully treated. The total success rate was 74% in a follow up after two years. Failure cases included 14 fenestrations with insufficient hearing gain, four fenestrations with secondary closure of the fistula and three fenestrations with labyrinthitis and deafness. Success of the operation depended on the post-operative course of a possible labyrinthitis serosa, caused among others by an inflammatory reaction of the flap over the created fenestra. To diminish this danger, Rüedi went back to the retro-aural two-stage fenestration as proposed by Sourdille.

In 1950, Cawthorne divided his patients at the first interview – so before the operation – into three groups:

- Suitable cases were patients with speech at conversational level: Unamplified: three inches; amplified: 12 feet; normal bone conduction;
- Borderline cases were patients with speech at conversational level: Unamplified: not heard; amplified: six feet; reduced bone conduction;
- Unsuitable cases were patients with speech at conversational level: Unamplified: not heard; amplified: four feet; profound reduced bone conduction.

Using this classification, Cawthorne suggested that suitable cases had 50% chance, borderline cases 30% chance and unsuitable cases 20% chance of long-term hearing improvement.

Lumsden (1958) also used pre-operative findings to classify patients into three groups: favorable, borderline or doubtful, and unfavorable. Favorable cases were patients in whom clinical and audiometric examination showed no appreciable degree of inner-ear deafness, while pure-tone audiometric examination by air conduction showed that hearing loss in the speech frequencies did not exceed 60 dB. Classified as borderline were cases in whom deafness was of such a degree that maximum improvement would be needed if serviceable or socially adequate hearing was to be the result. In pure-tone audiometric examination, the loss at one or more speech frequencies by air conduction could exceed

60 dB, but the loss in the speech frequencies by bone conduction (representing impairment of inner-ear function), after making the necessary corrections, did not exceed 30 dB. Unfavorable cases were patients in whom the associated inner-ear deafness was of such a degree that chances of success were practically nil. Net loss in speech frequencies by bone conduction exceeded 30 dB. The results of fenestration surgery were classified as successful when all three of the following criteria were met: 1) The patient was satisfied that serviceable or socially adequate hearing had been obtained; 2) The patient's ability to hear conversational voices and whispers was verified through tests; 3) Average hearing loss by air conduction in speech frequencies on the pure-tone audiometer did not exceed 30 dB at the end of a period of two to ten years following the operation. In a follow up of two to ten years after fenestration, Lumsden found that, applying these criteria to the group of patients classified as favorable, 79% of these cases could be considered successful, 10% of the cases showed improved hearing, in 7% hearing was unchanged and in 4% hearing was worse post-operatively. In the borderline group of patients these figures were respectively 20% successful, 57% improved, and 23% unchanged or worse. In the group of unfavorable cases 41% were rated successful or improved, while in 59% of the cases post-operative hearing was unchanged or worse.

In 1985, Brooks studied the long-term results of 25 years of follow up of the fenestration technique. The study included 58 patients who were operated on between 1953 and 1958. Adequate follow-up information was obtained of 28 of the original 58 subjects. Of these, three still had hearing above the social adequacy hearing level of 30 dB. Fifty percent of the subjects had hearing that was still significantly better than it had been prior to surgery. Twenty-five years after fenestration, more than 50% of the patients were using hearing aids, generally with a high degree of satisfaction.

Table 7 shows the results of fenestration as treatment for otosclerosis according to different authors.

Table 7. A collection of the hearing results after the fenestration surgery for otosclerosis by different ear surgeons.

Author	Year	# ptnts		Follow-up	Hearing improved	Comment
Sourdille	1935	109	Staged		74%	
Lempert	1938	23	One stage		80%	
Simpson-Hall	1944	66	Staged	6 years	66%	1 death
Garnett Passe	1946	170	Staged		60%	stopple
Simpson-Hall	1946	118	One stage		69%	stopple
Garson	1947	35	One stage	3 years	63%	conjuctiva
Lumsden	1949	21	Staged		66%	facial parese (2 cases)
Shambaugh	1949	2100	One stage	5 years	84%	
Lempert	1949	3700	One stage	6 years	74.4%	stopple
Jongkees	1949	100	One stage	1 year	78%	
Cawthorne	1950	198	One stage	3 years	50%-80%	removal stapes in 23 cases
Jongkees	1950	25	Popper	1 year	68%	
Meurman	1950	150	Popper	3 years	75.5%	
Shambough	1951	390	One stage		70%	
Garnett Passe	1951	611	One stage	3 years	70%	abandoned stopple
Rüedi *et al.*	1951	104	Staged	3½ years	74%	
Cawthorne	1953	200	One stage	6 years	75%	10% reclosure fenestra
Hunter	1954	51	Staged	1½ years	68%	
Poulsen	1954	140	Popper	2 years	50%	13 discharge
Lumsden	1958	139	One stage	2-10 years	79%	
Brooks	1985	28	One stage	25 years	50%	50% a hearing aid

3. Mobilization of the stapes and stapediolysis

3.1. Stapes mobilization

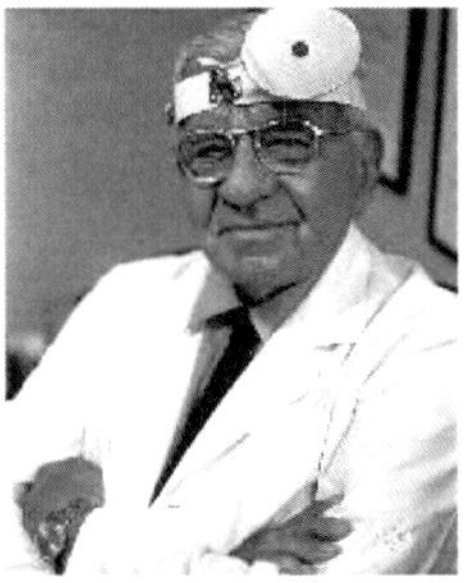

Fig. 73. Samuel Rosen.

Major medical discoveries sometimes appear to happen by accident, yet the real reason for what seems a miracle usually turns out to be the presence of a highly knowledgable scientist at the right place and time. To Samuel Rosen (1897-1981; Fig. 73), already a successful specialist in the Lempert fenestration operation, the patient's cry 'Oh Dr Rosen, I can hear you,' as Rosen tested the stapes for mobility, could have seemed an accident.

In 1952, Rosen published his first results after five ear surgeries in which he mobilized the fixated stapes prior to a fenestration operation. He realized that mobilization of the fixated stapes in otosclerosis could yield very good hearing results, perhaps even better than a fenestration. Furthermore, the surgical approach for a mobilization was much simpler than a fenestration. Rosen started performing this re-invented stapes mobilization on all of his otosclerosis patients and published the results in 1953. Oddly enough, Rosen did not mention past publications on mobilization of the stapes and stapedectomy performed by ear-surgery pioneers at the end of the 19th century. After this publication, Rosen was overwhelmed by otosclerosis patients who wanted his 'new' simple operation. Like Lempert fifteen years before, Rosen gave demonstrations of his surgical technique for otologists who were anxious to learn how to perform the operation.

The operation was conducted with local anaesthetic so that a hearing test could be carried out during the procedure. The incision was derived from that of Lempert (1946) for the tympanosympathectomy. It was made through the skin over the bony ear-canal wall, beginning at about nine o'clock and then continuing downward and around to three o'clock on the right ear, and vice versa on the left ear, about seven millimetres outward from the drum. The skin was then separated from the bone towards the tympanal membrane. The eardrum was lifted out of the sulcus and the middle ear was explored. In most cases, the incudo-stapedial junction was visible. To increase exposure, the edge of the posterior bony canal just external of the incus was removed. At that point, a good view was obtained of the incudo-stapedial joint, the stapes tendon, the chorda tympani nerve, the crura and the footplate of the stapes. To test the (im) mobility of the stapes footplate, a probe was placed against the upper part of the long process of the incus close to the articulation with the stapes. When the stapes was immobile, firm but controlled pressure was applied towards the inner ear. At that point, a normal stapes has its maximum movement and therefore it seemed logical to apply the pressure first in an effort to mobilize the otosclerotic bone. With pulsating pressure towards the oval window, the whole stapes was compressed from head to footplate in the inner ear. In early otosclerotic cases this approach was sufficient to mobilize the stapes. McKenzie and Rainer strongly suggested to attempt to rock the stapes from side to side in the axis of the long diameter of its footplate when this was insufficient. Rosen supported another mobilization manoeuvre: applying downward pressure on the footplate of the stapes anteriorly. All these attempts to mobilize the stapes in the oval window, however, could lead to fracturing of the stapedial crurae and in these cases Rosen performed a footplate fenestration with 'Gelfoam' dressing in the hole of the footplate. Rosen re-invented many special middle-ear instruments which were usable in combination with the new operation microscope. The Rosen-needles (Fig. 75) still are very useful instruments.

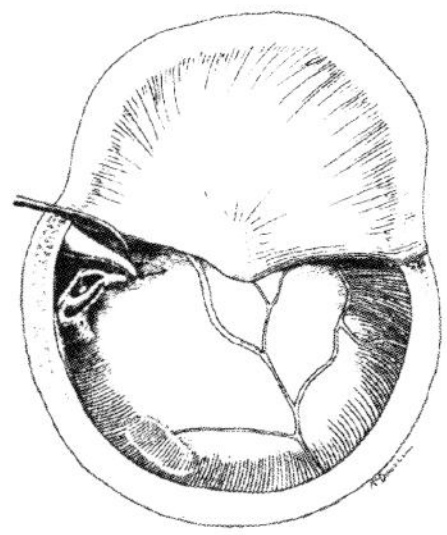

Fig. 74. Mobilization of the stapes described by Rosen.

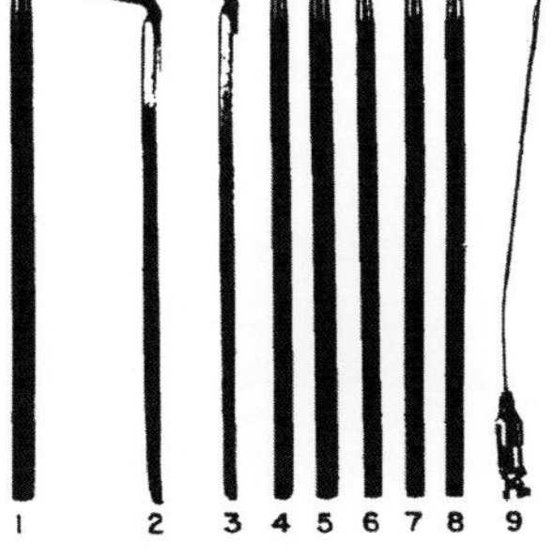

Fig. 75. Rosen's instruments, numbered in the order in which they are used in the mobilization of the stapes.

In 1954, Zollner reported that during a fenestration operation the 'posterior' crus of the stapes broke and that at the same time the footplate cracked in the middle. In his opinion this, and the fact that the footplate of the stapes does not heal following fracture, was the key to what really happened when Rosen's mobilization operation was successful for otosclerosis.

3.2. Stapediolysis

In Sweden, Holmgren started to perform Rosen's stapes mobilization method. He noticed that in a considerable number of cases it was not possible to avoid fracturing the stapes footplate. Holmgren, and later on Fowler, used a method in which the footplate was intentionally fractured (Fig. 76). After removal of the musculus stapedius for optimal view of the footplate, the posterior part of the footplate was mobilized by fracturing the middle part of the footplate close to the anteriorly fixated otosclerotic part. Figure 77 demonstrate the different steps of the stapediolysis as described by Holmgren.

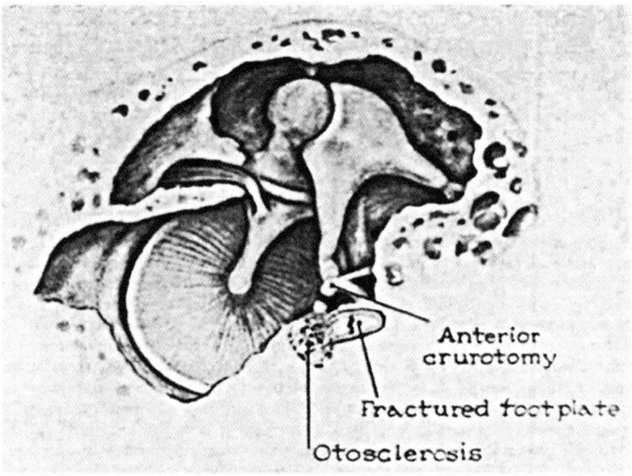

Fig. 76 (above). Drawing of Fowler's presentation of the stapediolysis.

The surgery was performed using local anaesthetic. At the moment of fracturing the footplate, patients often experienced a slight vertigo. When the footplate was fractured, perilymph well-up could be observed. At that stage of the operation, some patients noticed a change in hearing, apart from the vertigo.

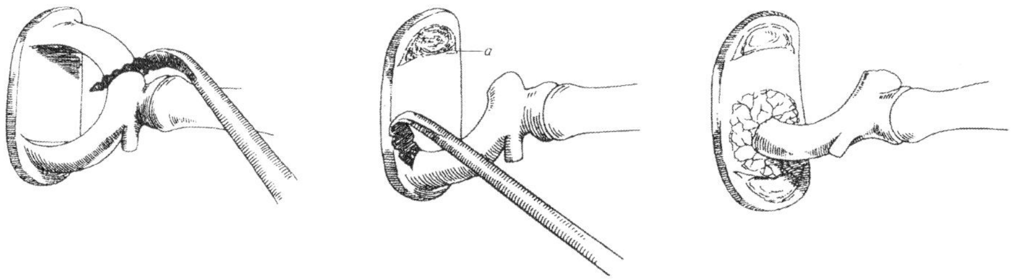

Fig. 77 (above). The different stages of Holmgren's mobilization and stapediolysis.

Occasionally a marked improvement in hearing was achieved in cases where the plate was thickened and sclerotic bone around the anterior attachment of the crus was found. The next step of the so-called stapediolysis was the cutting of the anterior crus of the fixated stapes suprastructure. By fracturing the anterior crus of the stapes, the posterior crus – still attached to the long process of the incus – became mobile and could be pushed a little bit into the cranial direction to form a 'new', mobile, one-crus stapes.

Although this procedure could be rather tricky because of anatomical variations and unexpected fractures, the results of stapediolysis were promising. In 1957, Frenckner designed a special instrument characterized as an automatic, oscillating chisel, which could be mounted on an ordinary dental drill to simplify fracturing of the anterior crus of the stapes during a stapediolysis.

In 1959, Juers published a procedure he called stapedioplasty. It was a modification of the stapediolysis technique introduced by Holmgren and Fowler in 1957. Juers invented the crurotomy saw to cut the anterior and posterior crus of the fixated stapes suprastructure in cases of otosclerosis (Fig. 78). Instead of breaking the middle part of the footplate, he fragmented the middle area of the fixated footplate after which the mobile posterior crus of the stapes arch was transported to the fragmented footplate at the point of optimum contact. Gelfoam was then placed around the transported crus to keep it in place and to prevent perilymph leakage.

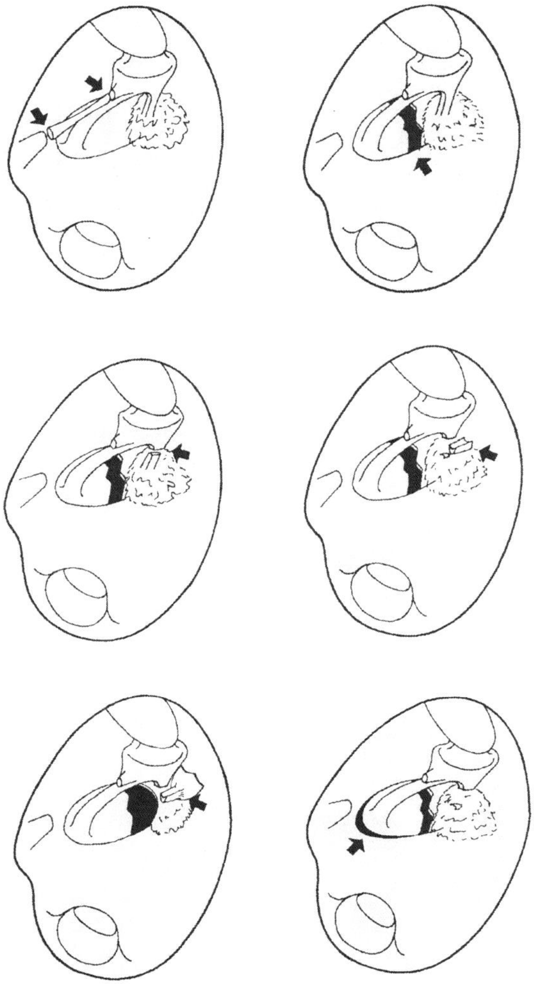

Fig. 78. The stapedioplasty with the microsaw according to Juers (1959).

For cases in which it was impossible to perform a stapes mobilization or a stapediolysis, Rüedi invented the so-called 'incudopexie' (1959; Fig. 79). After loosening the incus from the fixated stapes a fenestration of the horizontal semicircular was performed. Then the incus was remodelled and placed between the malleus head and into the fenestration, which was in turn covered by a vein graft. In total 172 such operations were performed by Rüedi in 1961 and a hearing gain of 10-60 dB was achieved in 58%. However, in 44% of these cases the gain disappeared completely

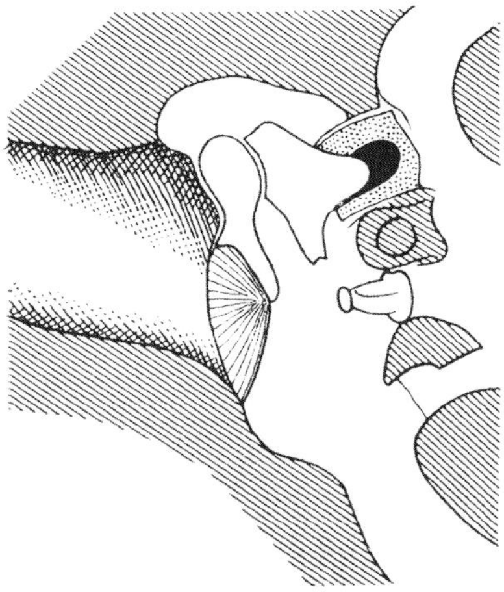

Fig. 79. Rüedi's incudopexie.

between one to three years after the operation, while in an additional 21% even a reduction in hearing occurred. Because so-called transmeatal fenestration of the horizontal semicircular canal by means of incudopexy had failed to show advantages, Rüedi relinquished his procedure. He switched to stapedectomy with placement of a venous graft and repositioning of a modified stapes.

Interestingly, more than forty years later, in 1998, Silverstein 'invented' the same stapediolysis technique. The only difference compared to the method described by Holmgren and Fowler in 1957 was the use of an HGM argon laser to vaporize the anterior crus and to fracture the footplate to make the posterior crus mobile. Silverstein preserved the stapedius tendon using a method he called laser stapedotomy minus prosthesis (laser STAMP). Like Lempert and Rosen, who also forgot to give credit to those who were the first to perform their specific surgical treatment of otosclerosis, Silverstein neglected to mention Holmgren's and Fowler's achievements in his publications' references.

Table 8 shows the hearing results of stapes mobilizations performed by different ear surgeons.

Table 8. Results of different surgeons who performed stapes mobilization for otosclerosis.

Stapes mobilization	Year	Patients	Hearing improved	Hearing unchanged
Skoog	1953	150	50%	50%
Meurman	1954	44	32%	68%
Meurman	1955	76	43%	57%
Meurman	1956	127	72%	28%
Sheer	1957	500	75%	25%
Venters	1958	90	70%	30%
Rosen	1958	254	77%	22%
Cawthorne	1958	200	72%	28%
Miles Foxen	1958	50	66%	33%
Gill	1958	146	72%	28%
Zollner	1959	140	75%	25%
Holmgren	1960	160	80%	20%

Naturally, older surgeons, who had been using the classic fenestration technique to treat otosclerosis all their lives, were rather critical about mobilization of the stapes and the stapediolysis technique. A leading American otologist (probably Lempert) called these new operations: *'orthopaedic-otological proletary surgery'* and he added: *'Something is broken apart without reason and without foreknowledge of the results. It is to be hoped that developments will rapidly lead to the time when such designation will no longer be justified'* (Frenckner, 1957).

Rambo, long-time partner of Lempert, endeavoured to create a bridge between the success of the stapes mobilization and the classic Lempert fenestration. He devised an alternative fenestration operation in which he approached the tympanic cavity through the usual mobilization incision, but raised a larger skin-flap than usual from the posterior meatal wall. He removed the bone from the Rivinian notch and extracted the incus. He then carefully dissected the malleus from the tympanic membrane and removed it. This step was necessary to make the tympanic membrane lie comfortably over the oval window. The stapes was then removed, after fragmentation if needed, and the tympanic membrane or skin-flap was laid over the oval window, invaginated into it and packed down. Rambo claimed that the fenestra ovalis now took the place of an opening in the external semicircular canal. The drum adhered to the promontory and an air-filled space remained in the hypotympanum with free communication between the Eustachian tube and the round window. This operation made a mastoidectomy and subsequent care of the cavity unnecessary. The fenestra ovalis, which is the natural route for the transmission of air-borne sound, should not tend to close or the result would be spoiled. This alternative fenestration approach was published just before the presentation of stapedectomy with interposition of a stapes prosthesis by Shea.

4. Stapedectomy and stapedotomy

4.1. Stapedectomy

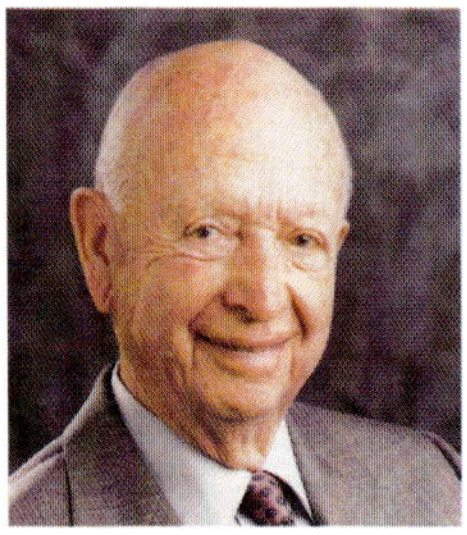

Fig. 80. Howard House.

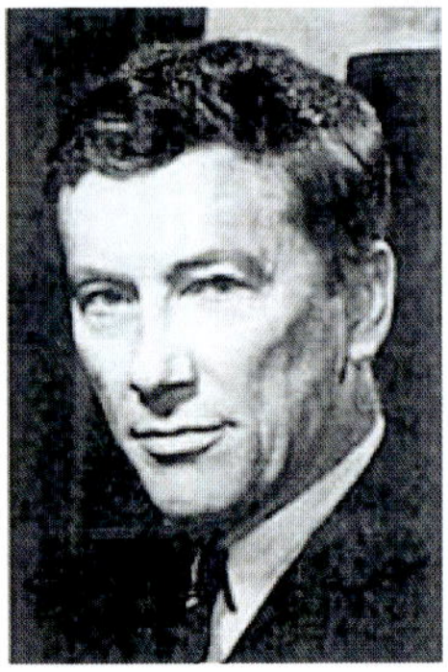

Fig. 81. John Shea.

In the 1950s, Rosen popularized the stapes mobilization technique by giving demonstrations of his surgical approach for otologists, with the aim of getting them to start using this new treatment of otosclerosis. Howard House (1908-2003; Fig. 80) was one of the first to practice this approach besides fenestration surgery. Another young otologist, John J. Shea (1924; Fig. 81), watched Rosen operate during one of his courses in the fall of 1953. Shea came to Los Angeles to be trained in fenestration surgery and stapes mobilization techniques by House in a one-month course. Instead of being there for just one month, however, he stayed in Los Angeles for six months.

House was impressed by the 'excellent surgical hands' of Shea and encouraged him a lot. One night, when the two were reviewing the day's surgery, Shea suggested House to take out the whole stapes and put something else in its place over or in the oval window. House had his reservations about this new idea of a stapes prosthesis. Shea encouraged House to enhance the idea and House replied: 'Any new idea is better than no idea and too many people have no ideas.' Shea left Los Angeles and started his own practice in Memphis.

Before Shea worked with House, he had lived in Europe for a while. In 1954, he had gone to study at the first ear clinic in Europe, located in Vienna and was founded by the famous Adam Politzer. There he had assisted in the operating room to become skilled at classic fenestration. In his spare time he had dissected fresh temporal bones to learn the mobilization technique. Spending weekends in the medical library, Shea had studied the papers of the pioneers of the first stapes surgeries in the 19th century. He was impressed by the 1902 work of Frederick L. Jack, reporting good results in a case of a double stapedectomy with a follow up of ten years. Shea realized that even in the pre-antibiotic era removal of the stapes was not necessarily fatal to the hearing or the patient, as was generally believed until then. He considered sealing of the oval window after extraction of the stapes very important.

In his Memphis practice, Shea continued to perform stapes mobilization for otosclerosis. He tried the method as described by Rambo, but without success. In 1955, Shea performed his first stapedectomy with interposition of a narrow rod of homograft cortical bone. This prosthesis was placed between the incus and the oval window, which was covered with a thin slice of subcutaneous connective tissue. The immediate hearing gain was remarkable. Unfortunately, the homograft was rejected after a while and the patient had to be fitted with a hearing aid. Shea concluded that the material used for the replacement of the extracted stapes in otosclerosis should be as biocompatible as possible. From a colleague in orthopedic surgery, Shea learned that Teflon® was an optimal product that was almost never rejected. Richards Manufacturing Company, Inc. in Memphis produced Teflon® and, after studying the shape of a number of stapes bones, RMC materials engineer Harry Treace created several stapes prostheses for Shea to use (Fig. 82).

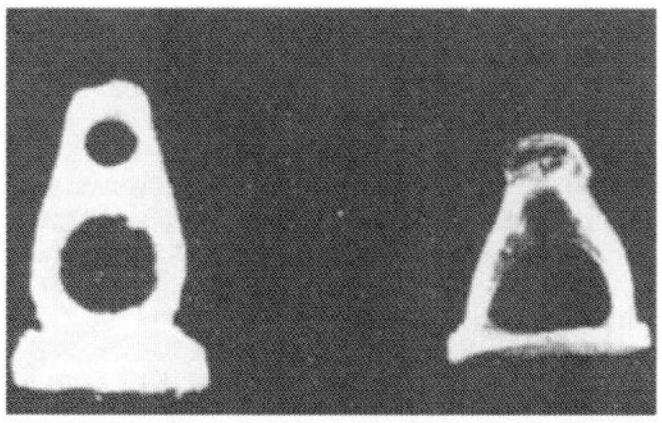

Fig. 82. The original Teflon® stapes prosthesis and a normal stapes.

On May 1, 1956, Shea performed a stapedectomy on a female patient, aged 54, and inserted a Teflon®-replica prosthesis onto the incus. The prosthesis rested on the oval window, which was covered by a graft on a prepared vein. The surgery was performed with local anaesthetic and the patient was able to hear better as soon as the implant was placed. After this successful stapedectomy with interposition of a stapes prosthesis, Shea continued performing this operation for otosclerosis.

In 1956, at the first Symposium on Mobilization of the Stapes at the Annual Triological Society meeting in Montreal, Shea showed his results to House, who suggested him to ask a question during the last presentation before lunch. House happened to be chairman of that session and he asked Shea to come to the podium to present his experience with this completely new concept in the treatment of otosclerosis. Shea presented his innovative work and House did not allow any comments from the audience in order to prevent heavy discussions and an inflamed attack on young Shea's work. This memorable presentation by Shea on May 17, 1956, can be considered to represent the most important change in the surgical treatment of otosclerosis. Stapedectomy with interposition of a stapes prosthesis became the new operation of choice for otosclerosis rather than mobilization of the stapes or fenestration of the lateral semicircular canal. The stapedectomy operation was to revolutionize otosclerosis surgery. At the Annual Triological Society meeting in San Francisco in 1958, Shea presented results of the first 89 patients who had been treated with a stapedectomy with vein graft and polyethylene tubing (Fig. 83). All showed good hearing improvement. At the same meeting, Schuknecht presented his results with the use of a stainless steel wire prosthesis to reconstruct the ossicular chain.

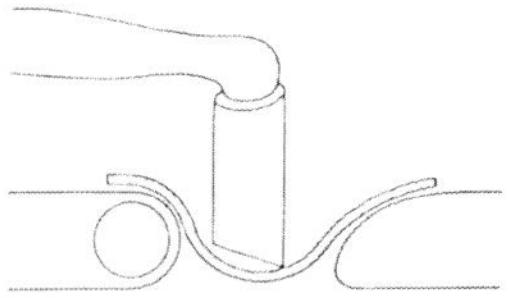

Fig. 83. Shea's classic stapedectomy with vein graft.

The new surgical approach for treating otosclerosis was the eclipse of Lempert. Stapedectomy became the treatment of choice among otologists and Lempert, who refused to use this new technique, noticed that the waiting list he had had for many years for his fenestration surgery shrank dramatically. His practice suffered and in the end he was forced to sell his hospital. In 1961, he moved into a small Manhattan office on 5th Avenue. He continued to perform fenestrations, but the stapedectomy procedure of Shea was superior. There was no need for his type of surgery anymore and his technique fell into oblivion. It was a painful experience for a surgical genius who had treated so many otosclerosis patients during more than twenty-five years. Lempert slowly slipped into a deep depression, followed by an early form of dementia. He was institutionalized in 1963 and died on December 14, 1968. House delivered the eulogy at the memorial service for the father of modern otiology.

Because of the reportedly excellent results of stapedectomy, this treatment became popular worldwide. Since Shea's development of the principle of stapedectomy for treating otosclerosis, numerous modifications have been described. These modifications were all based on the restoration of the sound conductive system using prosthetic material after complete or partial removal of the fixed stapes footplate. Portmann developed an interposition technique in which he displaced the anterior crus of the stapedial arch and removed most of the stapes footplate. The defect was covered with an autogenous vein graft on top of which the posterior crus was placed. Already in 1961, Goodhill from Los Angeles described various forms of the stapedectomy procedure. He distinguished between partial anterior crurectomy, hemistapedectomy, sub-total stapedectomy and total stapedectomy. As a natural follow up to stapediolysis as introduced by Holmgren in 1957, Causse (1964) developed the method of removal of the posterior part of the footplate with a vein graft and a Teflon®-piston interposition. Many of these stapedectomy variations are very well described by Tos, in his marvellous publication of 2000.

4.2. Small-hole stapedotomy

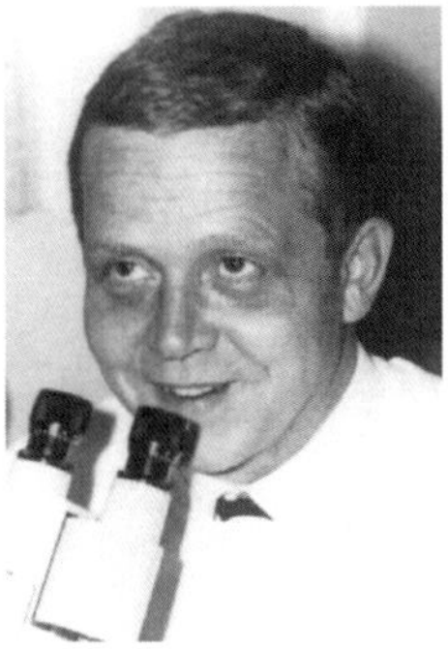

Fig. 84 (top). Jean Marquet.

In 1962, Shea *et al.* reported good results after making a small hole in the footplate and placing a Teflon®-piston without a vein graft. In 1963, Jean Marquet (1928-1991; Fig. 84) from Antwerp developed a modification of the surgical management of the stapes footplate. His work was published in 1965. He called his technique the platinotomy or the small-hole technique (Fig. 85). This technique was later called stapedotomy and developed excellent functional results. It also had a very low rate of sensorineural post-operative complications.

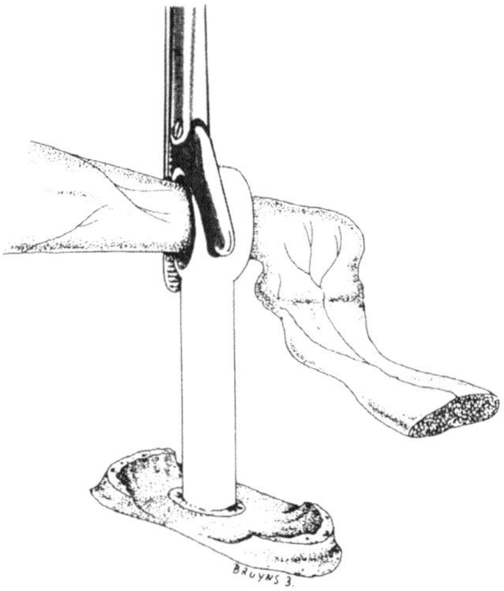

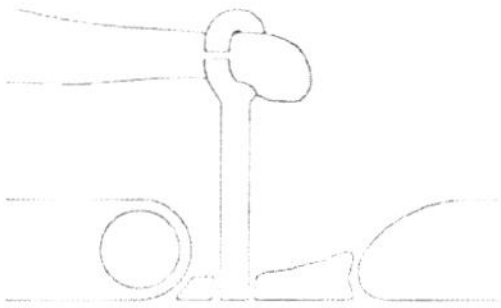

Fig. 85a & 85b (left & above). The stapedotomy as proposed by Jean Marquet.

The method consisted of the classic opening of the middle ear as developed by Rosen and exposure of the oval window area. The stapes suprastructure was separated from the long process of the incus, while the connection of the stapes muscle was kept intact, if possible. After removal of the stapedial arch, a pike was used to make a security perforation in the middle of the footplate. The security perforation hole was then enlarged using hooked micropikes, while leaving the annular ligament of the stapes footplate intact. A Teflon®-piston of 0.4 or 0.6 mm diameter was placed onto the incus and into the small hole of the stapes footplate. Marquet explicitly refused to perform his micro-hook technique with any kind of grafting material.

4.3. Laser stapes surgery

The focus for improving results of stapedotomy was on the creation of the small hole. The introduction of laser in otology by Perkins and DiBartolomeo in 1980 made it possible to make a small hole in the footplate (Fig. 86) without the risk of fracturing the whole footplate by manipulation with micro-hooks. Gantz *et al.* presented the first results of their small-hole stapedotomy with argon laser in 1982. A few years later, Palva demonstrated that results of stapedotomy with argon laser were slightly better in terms of hearing improvement than those of mechanical footplate perforation and reconstruction with wire and fascia. Gartner *et al.* studied the use of carbon dioxide (CO_2) laser in experiments on animals before this laser was introduced in the treatment of human ears by Lesinski *et al.* in 1989.

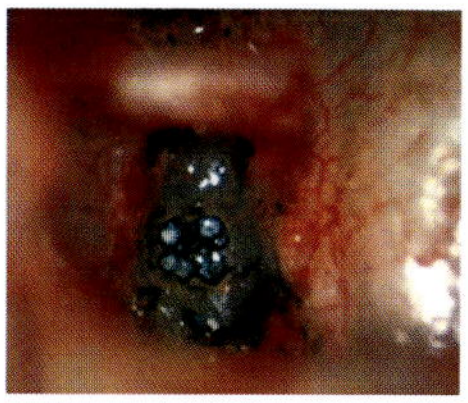

Fig. 86. A laser rosette to perforate the stapes footplate.

Table 9. Surgeons who introduced laser in stapes surgery.

Surgeon	Year	Laser stapedotomy
Perkins	1980	Argon
DiBartolomeo	1980	Argon
Gantz *et al.*	1982	Argon
McGee	1983	Argon
Gardner *et al.*	1984	CO2 animal study
Palva	1987	Argon
Silverstein *et al.*	1989	KTP
Lesinski *et al.*	1989	Argon, CO2 & KTP
Pfalz *et al.*	1992	Er.YAG
Strunck *et al.*	1993	Argon & KTP
Causse *et al.*	1993	Argon endo-otoprobe
Jovanovic *et al.*	1995	Nd:YAG, Er:YAG and CO2

The main advantages of laser stapedotomy were less vertigo, excellent hearing results and shorter hospital stays, as noted by McGee. In 1993, Gherini and Causse introduced the handheld-needle-probe fiberoptic argon laser to locally vaporize very tiny holes in the footplate. Table 9 shows the list of stapes surgeons who introduced different types of laser for the surgical treatment of otosclerosis.

Using a micro-drill, these tiny holes were then combined to create one hole with a diameter of about 0.8 mm. Because of the size of the hole, Causse needed a classical vein graft which he took from the hand. This classic method still is the treatment of choice in the famous Clinique du Docteur Jean Causse in Béziers, France. A modification of the stapedotomy technique was described by Fish (1994). He used an endaural approach and middle-ear exploration to carry out a small fenestration of the fixed stapes footplate with a manual perforator, followed by an interposition of his Teflon®-platinum prosthesis. These steps were followed by division of the incudostapedial joint and removal of the stapes suprastructure. However, the results of this technique did not exceed those of removal of the stapes crurae before stapedotomy and sometimes the technique was difficult to perform in cases of a narrow oval niche or a dehiscent overhanging facial nerve.

Nowadays, the suprastructure of the fixed stapes in otosclerosis is removed by using micro hooks and a crura nipper with or without a laser. Another modification of classic stapedectomy and stapedotomy was the preservation of the stapes tendon. In 1966, Girgis already described a technique to keep the stapes tendon intact in stapes surgery. Colletti (1988) applied the same technique as Girgis, but used a micro-drill. A later follow-up study reported this technique's good results. Causse invented a technique to reconstruct the stapes tendon, aiming to re-create the stapes reflex and thus prevent excessive movement of the implanted stapes prosthesis. After positioning a special stapes-piston with a platform near the loop, the reconstructed stapes tendon was placed on this platform and fixed with added fibrous tissue. Results of this method were published in one paper only and this technique has not been used in modern stapes surgery.

4.4. Stapes prostheses

Ever since Shea invented the stapes prosthesis, many different types of prostheses have been produced. Shea started with a Teflon® stapes-replica of the stapes and then moved on to a pointed polyethylene tube. Schuknecht adapted Shea's work and started using a stainless-steel wire as prosthesis. A piece of wire was bent to form a shepherd's crook and hooked on the long process of the incus. On its other side a piece of fat was fixed and positioned in the oval window after stapedectomy. Goodhill (1960) designed all kinds of differently modified and shaped polyethylene struts as stapes prostheses. Shea returned to using Teflon® in 1962 and he designed an entire fluoroplastic loop-prosthesis with a shaft of 0.6 mm in diameter. In 1964, he invented the Teflon®-cup prosthesis (Fig. 87), which had a loop holding down the incus in the cup at the head of the prosthesis.

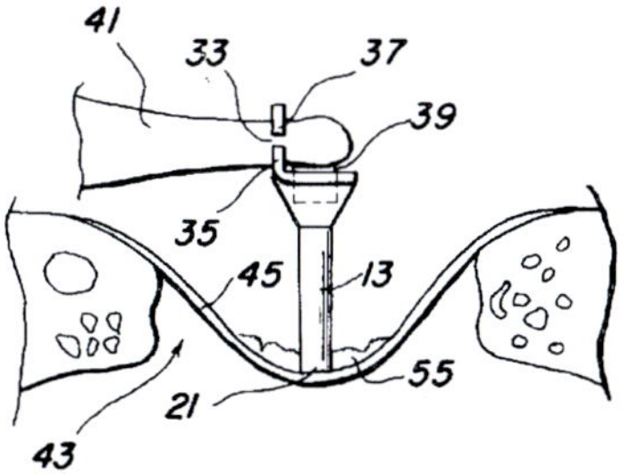

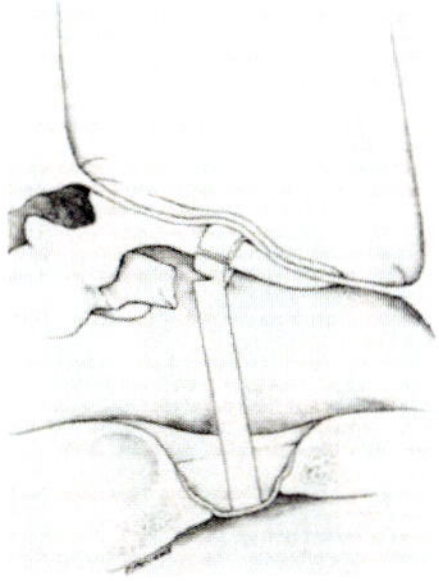

Fig. 87 (left). The Teflon® cup stapes prosthesis developed by Shea.

Fig. 88 (right). The Teflon® malleus attachment prosthesis for revision stapes surgery developed by Shea.

Shea developed a special malleus handle attachment prosthesis for revision cases in which the long process of the incus was necrotized (Figs. 88 & 89).

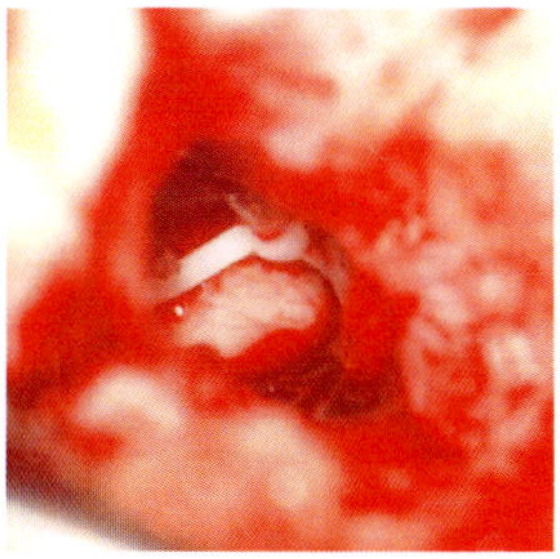

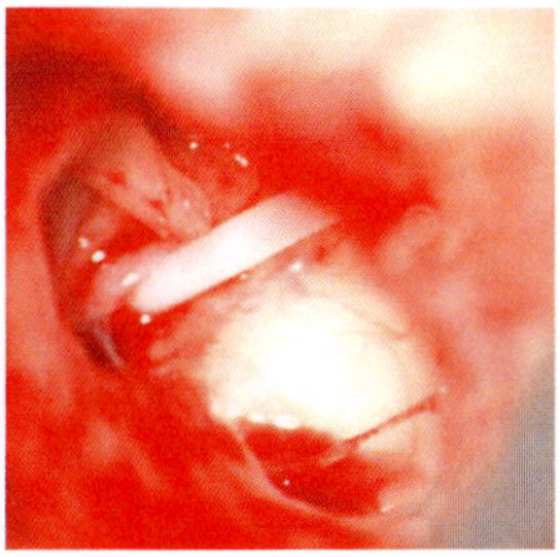

Fig. 89a & 89b. Shea's malleus attachment prosthesis on the malleus (left) and into the small fenestra of the footplate (right) bypassing the atrophic incus.

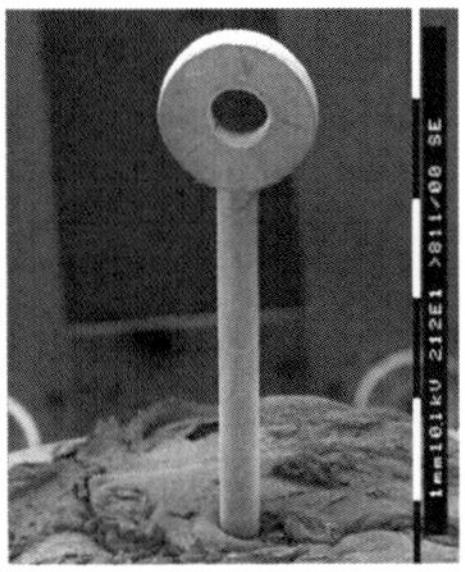

Fig. 90. Scanning electron microscope (SEM) image of Causse Teflon® loop piston.

Causse and Cawthorne designed modifications of the Shea Teflon® loop-prosthesis, altering the diameter of the shaft (Fig. 90). At the end of the 1960s, wire-plastic stapes pistons were introduced. De La Cruz designed a platinum-fluoroplastic piston with a shortened piston shaft to increase visibility while placing it. Fish designed a platinum-fluoroplastic piston with a flat, ribbon-like loop. Modifying the Teflon®-cup designed by Shea, pistons with stainless-steel cups and bucket-handles were invented. In 1992, Pusalkar and Steinbach introduced gold as a material for a stapes prosthesis. The pure-gold piston, on the market since 1995 (Fig. 91), yielded very good results in hearing improvement, often showing an overclosure of bone-conduction thresholds.

However, the golden stapes prosthesis was taken off the market after eight years, as a result of a few cases of reparative granuloma, considered to have been possibly caused by a reaction to this piston. In 1999, a new rigid and low-weight titanium stapes piston entered the market (Fig. 92).

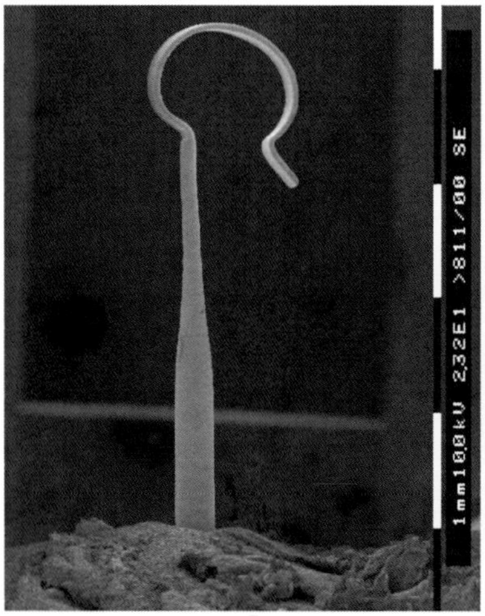

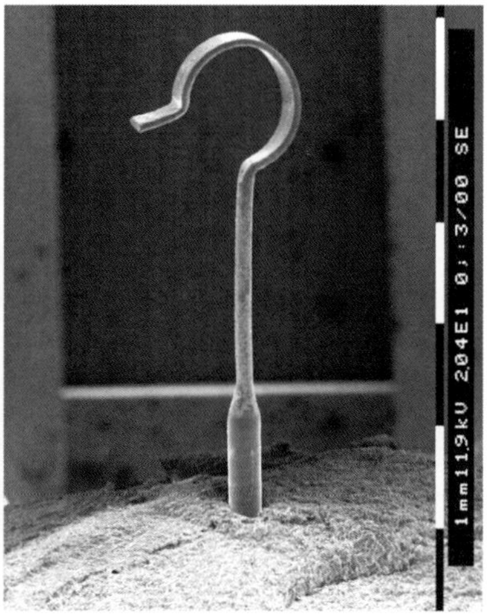

Fig. 91 (left). SEM image of the golden K-piston.

Fig. 92 (right). SEM image of Titanium K-piston.

Zuur *et al.* *(2003)* demonstrated that this so-called titanium K-piston was also successful in restoration of hearing after stapedotomy. Kwok *et al.* *(2002)* showed in a comparative SEM study that the titanium prosthesis could be considered the most suitable prosthesis for stapes surgery. The attachment of the stapes prosthesis onto the incus became a subject of interest in the beginning of the twenty-first century. À Wengen (2003) designed a new, self-retaining titanium-clip stapes prosthesis (Fig. 93), which did not encircle the long process of the incus (Fig. 94). The unique design of this prosthesis allegedly reduced the risk of incus necrosis and it was also seen as an advantage of the clip-piston that it required no crimping onto the incus.

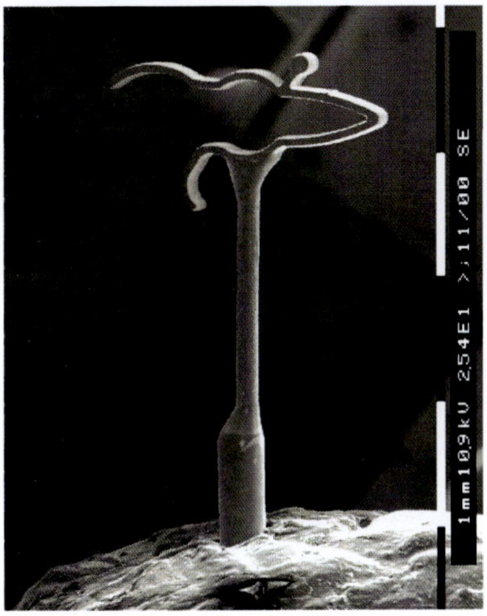

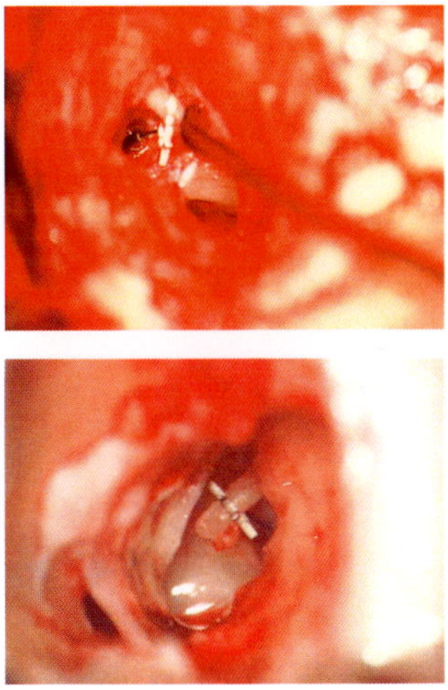

Fig. 93 (left). SEM image of the titanium à Wengen clip piston.

Fig. 94 (right). A Wengen clip piston onto the long process of the incus.

In 2005, Knox introduced a stapes prosthesis with a Nitinol wire-loop and a Teflon® shaft: the SMart-piston prosthesis. The prosthesis is provided in an open conformation, but in its closed position it is designed to crimp firmly around the long process of the incus. After the loop of the prosthesis is appropriately positioned over the long process of the incus, a transition from open to closed position is induced by the application of a heat source (mini-bipolar or laser) with a temperature of 45°C. Therefore, no manual crimping is necessary for this process. A recent comparative study demonstrated that use of the SMart-piston prosthesis results in air-bone gap closure similar to that of the classic platinum-fluoroplastic piston, but offers the added advantage of reduced surgery time. A so-called Soft Clip titanium piston was recently (2007) introduced as successor for the à Wengen clip piston. The advantage of this new piston is that it needs 40% less force to clip the prosthesis on the incus compared to the à Wengen clip piston. The first reported hearing results achieved with the Soft Clip are promising. However, a longer follow-up study is needed for conclusions to be drawn. The latest development in stapes prostheses is the NiTiBOND® stapes prosthesis. This prosthesis combines the clip-stapes design with the shape memory effect of Nitinol. The piston is made of pure titanium, except for the Nitinol-loop. A flat-band Nitinol-loop with contact-free zones diffuses the impact of pressure on the incus. When heat is applied by laser to the contact-free zones on the loop, the shape memory properties of Nitinol cause the loop to close. The contact-free zones function as thermal blockers, limit heat dispersion on the mucosa and minimize the risk of incus and mucosa strangulation. Preliminary short-term results suggest the new NiTiBOND® stapes prosthesis is safe and reliable (Huber *et al.* 2011), although in the author's experience hearing results are the same compared to all other, older types of stapes prostheses. Table 10 shows a collection of data on some hearing results of stapededotomies during the first decade of the 21st century. In table 11 the general average hearing results over eighty years of the surgical treatment of otosclerosis are presented

Table 10. Results of stapes surgery.

	Year	#	Hearing improved	Hearing unchanged	Hearing loss
Kos *et al.*	2001	604	89%	?	?
Gurgel *et al.*	2002	59	90%	5%	5%
Freitas *et al.*	2006	51	92.1%	5.9%	2.0%
Song *et al.*	2006	39	92.3%	?	?
Marchese *et al.*	2007	212	93%	?	5-8.03%
Booncho *et al.*	2007	109	92.5%	7,5%	?
Kisilevsky *et al.*	2009	1145	94.5%	5%	0,5%
Vincent *et al.*	2009	3050	94.2%	5.3%	0.5%
Tange (recent data)	2013	1345	93.9%	5.2%	0.9%

Table 11. Results of surgical treatment of otosclerosis over more than 80 years.

	Year	Hearing improved	Hearing unchanged	Hearing loss
Fenestration	1930-1952	70%	25%	5%
Stapes mobilization	1952-1958	65%	35%	-
Stapedectomy	1956-	94%	5%	1%

Chapter five

Treatment of cochlear otosclerosis

1. Histology on cochlear otosclerosis

Otosclerotic deposits, not associated with hearing loss, are found in approximately 10% of all adult temporal bones, as autopsies of caucasian people have shown. Otosclerosis is a common focal lesion of the otic capsule of unknown aetiology. It is found principally in relation with the cochlea and footplate of the stapes. Cochlear otosclerosis is defined as otosclerosis located in the otic capsule involving the cochlear endosteum. It causes sensorineural hearing loss and often also a mixed-type hearing loss. It has been clearly shown that when otosclerosis is so severe that it involves the cochlear endosteum, it usually fixes the stapes as well. This expression of otosclerosis in or around the cochlea was already observed by otologists in the beginning of the 20th century. Siebenmann (1911), Manasse (1912), Mayer (1928; Fig. 95) and, later, Nager and Fraser (1938; Fig. 96) conducted histological examinations of temporal bones of patients with severe otosclerosis.

Fig. 95. Histological drawing of Mayer (1928) of otosclerosis involving the cochlea (A).

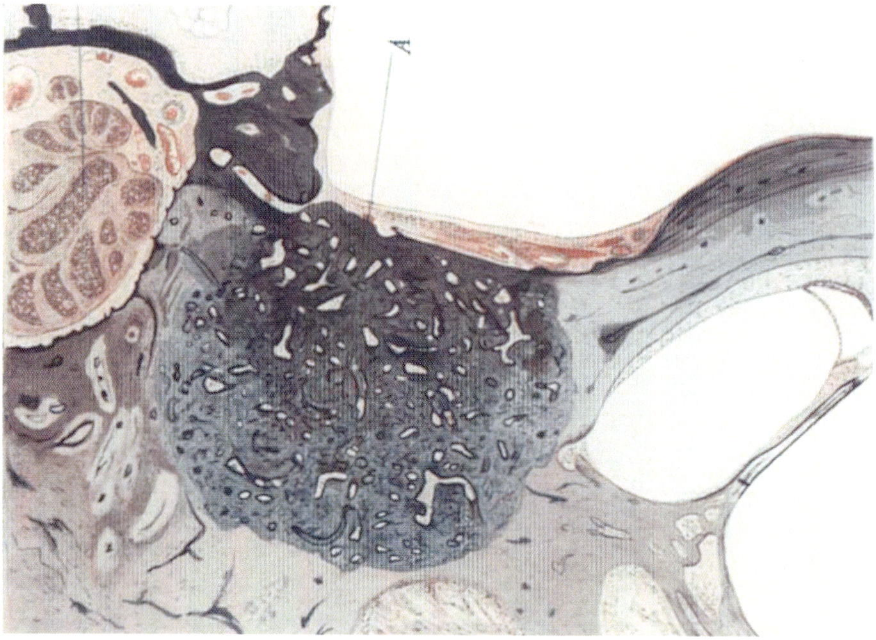

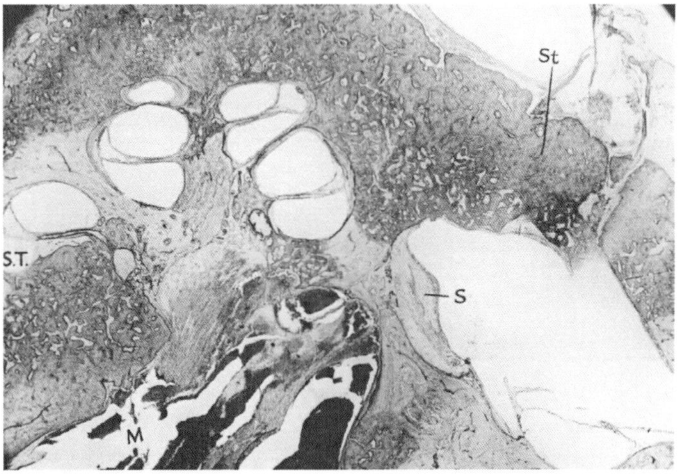

Fig. 96 (right). Nager's histology of a severe case of cochlear otosclerosis (St = stapes footplate; S = succulus; S.T. = otosclerosis in scala tympani).

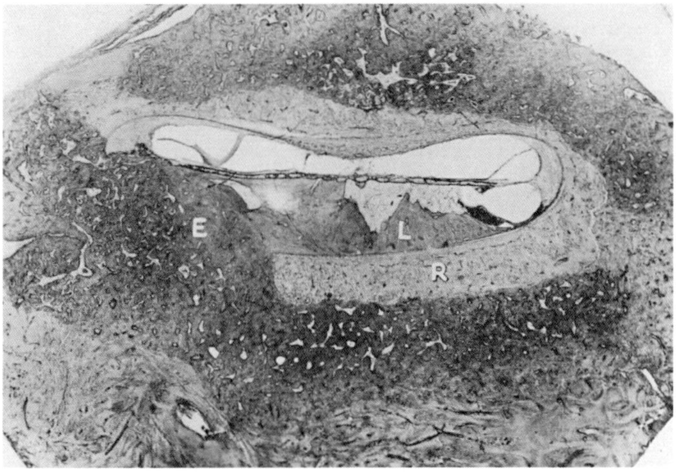

Fig. 97 (left). Otosclerosis in scala tympani 1938.

These examinations clearly showed the newly-formed otosclerotic bone tissue penetrating the scala tympani (Fig. 97). Occurrence of this 'aggressive' type of otosclerosis was believed to be about 5% of normal otosclerosis cases (Bosatra, 1960).

Histopathologic confirmation of cochlear otosclerosis was demonstrated by Rüedi (1966). He observed circumscribed swellings of the stria vascularis in the region of the active otosclerotic focus in temporal bones of 37 patients with otosclerotic fixation of the stapes. In five cases of otosclerosis with fairly severe perceptive hearing loss, obvious inner-ear changes were found, like lamellar new bone formation and atrophy of the inner ear. In all of these cases circumscribed swellings of the stria vascularis were also manifest. Holleman and Harrill (1967) and Sando *et al.* (1968) also observed solitary cochlear otosclerosis in their studies of temporal bone case. Linthicum *et al.* (1978), supported by the observations of Rüedi, proposed that an enzymatic concept of otospongiosis could explain the most important part of the sensorineural impairment in cochlear otospongiosis. Through micro-dissection and surface preparations of otosclerotic temporal bones, Hawkins *et al.* (1978) demonstrated that severe sensorineural degeneration was associated with large otosclerotic foci that reached all the cochlear turns. It was postulated that possibly a toxic factor diffused from the otosclerotic focus and acted directly on the organ of Corti. In addition, extensive active capsular otosclerosis resulting in severe sensorineural degeneration of the vestibular system was described. In a renewed study of his temporal-bone collection, Schuknecht (1979) concluded that sensorineural hearing loss without associated conductive loss could not be attributed to otosclerosis. He stated that in cases when the otosclerotic lesion was so severe as to cause damage to the organ of Corti there must always be fixation of the stapes.

2. Radiological investigation for cochlear otosclerosis

In 1979, Schuknecht doubted the reliability of polytomographic radiology methods to diagnose otosclerosis. At the same time, Freeman (1979) used data out of his private practice to show that a high percentage of diagnostic problems are due to cochlear otosclerosis. The diagnosis of otosclerosis was clinically supported roentgenologically. Balle and Linthicum (1984) demonstrated that in many cases of cochlear otosclerosis only sensorineural hearing loss could be present, without stapedial fixation. They postulated that many cases of cochlear otosclerosis might go undiagnosed. Patients with progressive sensorineural hearing loss and a family history of otosclerosis could be assumed to have cochlear otosclerosis. Polytomographic research helped diagnose cochlear otosclerosis. Since 1963, enormous work on the imaging of cochlear otosclerosis has been performed by Valvassori, starting with imaging of otosclerotic temporal bones. In a CT-scan research, Swartz *et al.* (1985) were able to correlate audiometrical data of sensorineural hearing loss in otosclerosis with CT findings and with involvement of the frequency level subtended by the specific area of the cochlea involved. Cochlear involvement of otosclerosis is most frequent in elderly patients, but can also occur in children. Havriliak and Parisier (1991) presented a case of cochlear otospongiosis in a 14-year-old child. A CT scan demonstrated changes characteristic of otosclerosis. The patient had a strong family history of otosclerosis and showed mild-to-moderate sensorineural hearing loss with stapes reflexes being absent. Radiological investigation of temporal-bone lesions acquired importance after the invention of Computed Tomography (CT) in 1972, and especially after introduction of high-resolution CT (HRCT) and multi-slice CT (MSCT) in 1978 by Valvassori. Recently, Yongkang Ou *et al.* (2009) reported on patients mainly complaining of recurrent episodic vertigo or equilibrium disturbance together with progressing hearing loss. The characteristics shown in HRCT scanning were: low-density areas in different areas of the otic capsule with pericochlear lucency or double-ring effect as typical signs of cochlear otosclerosis (Figs. 98 & 99). They concluded that HRCT scanning of the temporal bone plays an important role in the clinical diagnosis of cochlear otosclerosis. Abou Seree *et al.* (2011) also confirmed that HRCT scans are a very valid tool that can be used to confirm, localize, and determine the size of clinically suspected otosclerotic foci. Cases classified as doubtful or negative pre-operatively should alert surgeons to the possibility of intra-operative complications and/or post-operative sensorineural hearing loss.

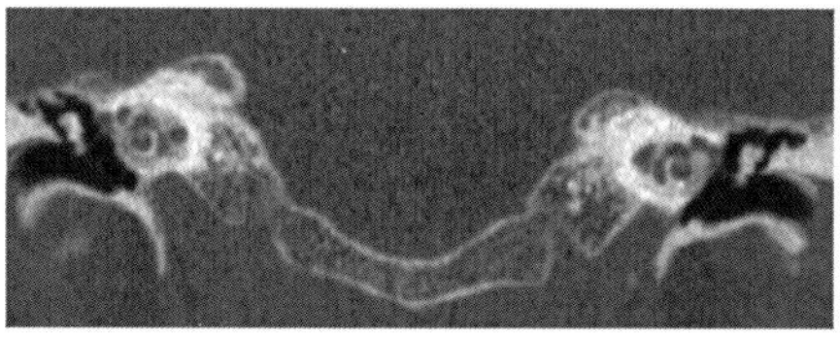

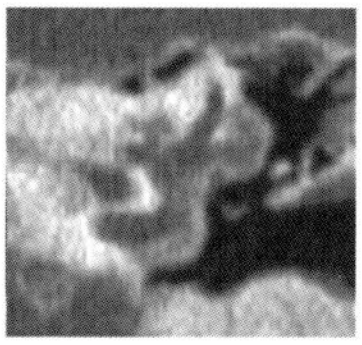

Fig. 98 (left). CT-scan of a case of cavitating cochlear otosclerosis.

Fig. 99 (right). CT-scan of cochlear otosclerosis involving the horizontal semicircular canal.

3. Treatment of sensorineural deafness due to cochlear otosclerosis

As described in Chapter 2, many different ways have been tried to stop the progression of sensorineural deafness in cases where the disease involved the cochlea. Local treatments, treatment with sex hormones, cortisone therapy or fluoride have all proven unsuccessful. X-ray treatment and the use of re-education machines did not stop the otosclerosic process in the cochlea. None of the alternative therapies managed to alter the progression of inner-ear deafness. In contrast, the success of surgical treatment of otosclerosis led to many patients with local fenestral otosclerosis being treated successfully. When the inner ear is involved in the otosclerotic process of sensorineural hearing loss, this hearing loss can progress notwithstanding a perfect surgical closure of the air-bone gap by a stapedotomy. When this process is rapid in its progression and total deafness comes into view, there is now fortunately the option of a cochlear implantation. This treatment of cochlear otosclerosis depends on the degree of sensorineural deafness. Brøndbo *et al.* (1983) discovered from their histological studies on temporal bones that there appeared to be two growth patterns of otosclerotic lesions. The first pattern showed an otosclerotic lesion growing for a very short period and then becoming dormant or inactive. The second pattern showed continuing growth of the lesion and progression throughout life. In cochlear otosclerosis, even after successful stapes surgery, the progression of sensorineural hearing impairment can be fast or slow, depending on the extensiveness of inner-ear involvement. In the beginning, a conventional hearing aid will suffice to manage the effects of cochlear otosclerosis. As the patient ages, however, the level of hearing impairment will exceed the power of hearing aids alone. In well-advanced cochlear otosclerosis as was first described by House and Sheehy in 1962, speech discrimination will decrease and conventional hearing aids are not effective anymore. Sound amplification will fail in these cases and cochlear implantation becomes a potential management option for those patients with far-advanced cochlear otosclerosis. The diagnosis far-advanced otosclerosis refers to patients suffering from a long-term otosclerosis with an air-conduction threshold of 85 dB or worse and a non-measurable bone-conduction threshold. This threshold's not being measurable is due to limitations of (current) audiometric equipment.

4. Cochlear implantation in far-advanced cochlear otosclerosis

Good results of cochlear implantation in cases diagnosed with far-advanced otosclerosis have been reported by Rama-López *et al.* (2006). Thirty cases that were diagnosed with cochlear otosclerosis, based on pericochlear hypodensities found using HRCT scans, showed CID sentence test improvement from 32% pre-implantation compared to 72% after three years of follow up. No complications related to the surgery itself, such as facial-nerve stimulation, were documented. They stated that cochlear implantation provided patients suffering from far-advanced otosclerosis with a good prognosis that is comparable to patients without cochlear otosclerosis. Rotteveel *et al.* (2004) on the other hand, studied the results of 53 patients with severe retrofenestral (cochlear) otosclerosis that had received implants. The patients were treated in four different cochlear implant centers in the United Kingdom and the Netherlands. They concluded that cochlear implant surgery in far-advanced otosclerosis can be challenging. They found a relatively high number of partial insertions and misplacements of the electrode array, for which revision surgery was needed. A very high proportion of patients experienced facial-nerve stimulation, mainly caused by the distal electrodes. They recommended to discuss this side-effect with patients pre-operatively. Morawiec-Bajda and Durko (2000) described benign paroxysmal position vertigo in cases of far-advanced cochlear otosclerosis. A treatment consisting of cochlear implantation and occlusion of the posterior semicircular canal as described by Parnes and McClure (1991) could accomplish good hearing results and could be effective in the management of vertigo as well (Crossland *et al.* 2004). Iurato *et al.* (1992) proposed the term 'very far-advanced otosclerosis' for otosclerotic patients with non-measurable air- and bone-conduction thresholds on a standard clinical audiometer, resulting in a blank audiogram. Calmels *et al.* (2007) studied patients with very far-advanced otosclerosis who received a stapedotomy or cochlear implantation and concluded that both objective and subjective results were statistically better in the cochlear implant group than in the stapedotomy group. Recently, Merkus *et al.* (2011) designed an algorithm built on an evidence-based strategy to facilitate decision-making in cases of advanced otosclerosis. Three parameters – speech performance, CT-scan classification and the extent of hearing loss – guide the surgeon to either a cochlear implantation, stapedotomy or hearing aid. Tange *et al.* (2009) advised to indicate a bilateral cochlear implantation in cases of far-advanced cochlear otosclerosis, because of the obliterative progression of the disease inside the inner ear (Figs. 100 & 101). This could lead to a situation where insertion of the cochlear electrode would become almost impossible. Nowadays, cochlear implantation is the treatment of choice in cases of far-advanced cochlear otosclerosis.

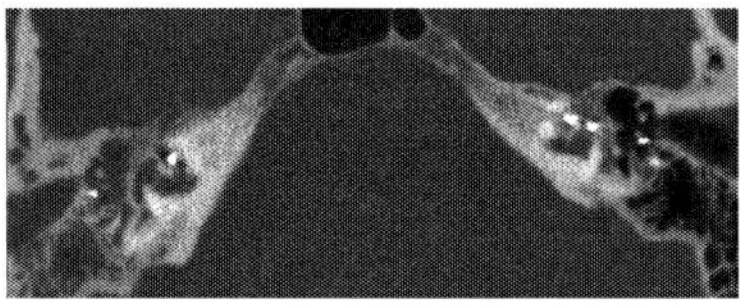

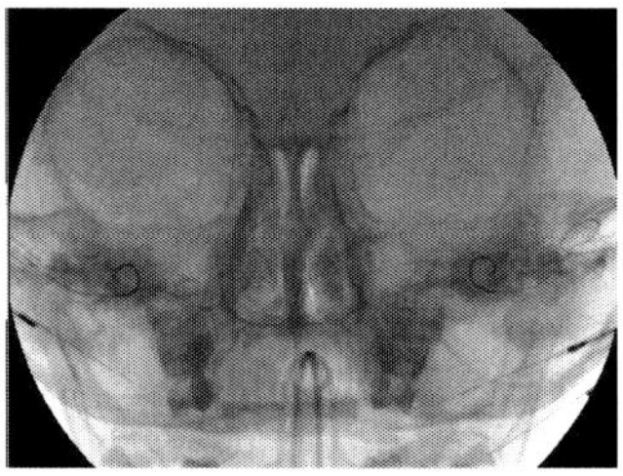

Fig. 100 (left). Bilateral cochlear implantation in a case of cochlear otosclerosis.

Fig. 101 (right). Per-operative radiography of bilateral cochlear implantation.

Final remarks

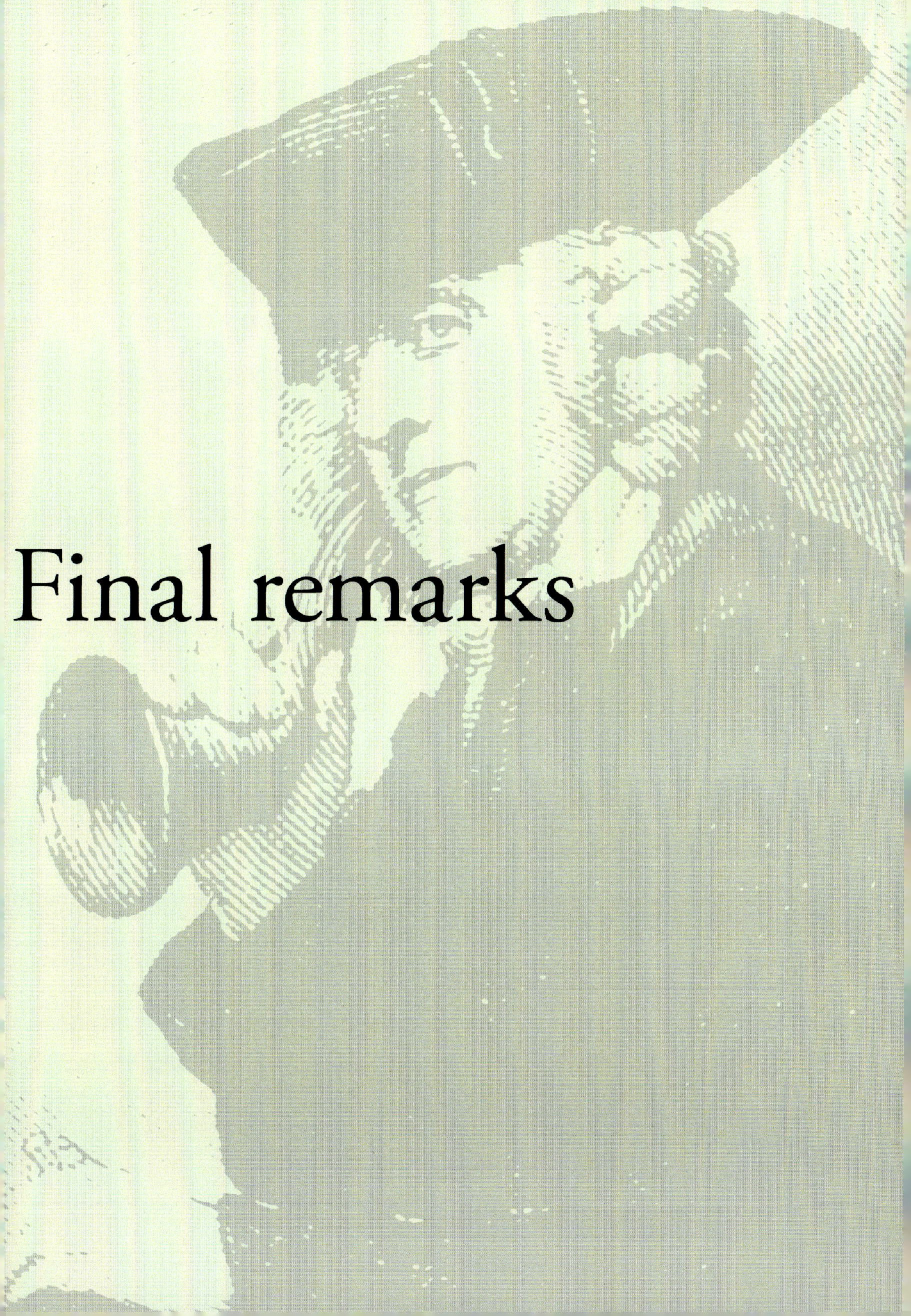

Final remarks

For as long as mankind exists, diseases have been a part of life. The development of knowledge of different diseases and their treatments forms part of our history. The history of knowledge on loss of hearing due to the disease now known as otosclerosis covers a relatively short period of time in the existence of mankind. After the discovery of the middle-ear structures in the 16th century, it took almost three centuries to discover the pathological origin of the fixation of the stapes in some cases of hearing loss. Temporal-bone studies demonstrated the pathology of fixated stapes and bone changes around the inner ear. The disease was initially called otospongiosis, but later on this name was changed to the more popular name otosclerosis. From the moment the origin of otosclerosis was known, all kinds of attempts have been made to treat this disease. Oto-massage of the drum was applied, aiming to mobilize the middle-ear chain. Surgical treatment, such as mobilization or extraction of the stapes, was followed by fenestration of the labyrinth. Unfortunately, successful results turned out to be only temporary, and in some cases treatment even caused fatalities as a result of serious infections. In 1900, leading otologists abandoned surgical treatment of otosclerosis and for more than a decade after that only conservative treatment was available. Medical treatment of thyroid and parathyroid glands was applied with moderate success. Re-education machines were invented to treat deafness and otosclerosis. After the discovery of X-rays these were also used as alternative treatment to cure otosclerosis. In cases of otosclerosis in pregnant females abortion and sterilization were sometimes performed to prevent further hearing loss and, in line with eugenic standards, also to avoid hearing-impaired offspring. The development of the surgical microscope, in the second decade of the 20th century, preluded a rebirth of surgical treatment for otosclerosis. Fenestration of the semicircular canals became the treatment of choice for more than twenty years. Fenestration led to far better results in hearing improvement than all conservative treatments. Sex hormone, thyroid, parathyroid and corticoid treatments were abandoned. Accidentally, mobilization of the stapes as treatment for fixated stapes in otosclerosis was reinvented in the early fifties. Results of that treatment were significantly better than those of classic fenestration. Unfortunately, in most cases fixation of the stapes recurred. Extracting the stapes and inserting a prosthesis finally proved to be the solution to overcome the problem of fixated stapes in otosclerosis. For over a century, otologists have been trying to find the optimal treatment of otosclerosis. In their struggle, all kinds of medical and surgical treatments and all kinds of devices have been applied. Most of these treatments are now considered obsolete or even bizarre. Still, these treatments have been at the basis of current, successful treatment of otosclerosis.

Table 12 gives an overview of most of the treatments trying to improve the hearing in otosclerosis since the discovery of the disease.

Future developments will likely diminish all possible side effects of surgical treatment. Research into the onset of the disease and the genetic factors involved will probably further refine treatment strategies. The role of cochlear involvement in the otosclerotic process and treatment to arrest that process, while keeping perceptive hearing intact, will be the main challenge for future research into the treatment of otosclerosis.

Table 12. An overview of most of the treatments for otosclerosis since the discovery of the disease.

Year	Authors	Surgical treatment	Medical treatment	Other treatments
1875	Mach	Stapes mobilization		
1876	Kessel	Stapes extraction		
1879	Rhodes			Audiphone
1880	Graydon			Dentaphone
1884	Lucae	Malleus mobilization		
1896	Anderston	Perforation stapes footplate		
1897	Passow	Window in the cochlea		
1899	Floderus	Fistula in lateral canal		
1899	Delstanche			Oto-massage
1900	Politzer, Siebenmann			Condemned stapes surgery for otosclerosis
1910	Bárány	Posterior canal fenestration		
1912	Manasse		Thyroid extracts	
1912	Maurice			Kinesiphone
1913	Zünd Burguet			Zünd-Burguet
1913	Ortloff			X-ray treatment
1913	Jenkins	Horizontal SCC fenestration		
1918	Blohmke			Artificial abortus
1925	Mirvish		Parathormone injections	
1928	Leicher	Parathyroid transplantation		
1929	Watson-Williams		Parathyroid tablets	
1929	Sourdille	Fenestration in two tempi		

Year	Authors	Surgical treatment	Medical treatment	Other treatments
1933	Wittmaack & Rollin	Raising up dura mater		
1935	Gray		Local Thyroxin	
1936	Alonzo & Chiarino	Parathyroidectomy		
1938	Lempert	One-stage fenestration		
1939	Bernstien & Gillis		Sex hormones	
1946	Popper	Endaural fenestration		
1950	Bordes-Valls	Neurosurgical fenestration		
1951	Riskaer		Corticothropin i.m.	
1952	Goodhill		Oral cortisone	
1952	Rosen	Stapes mobilization		
1954	Hutchinson		Local cortisone	
1956	Shea	Stapedectomy – Teflon® prosthesis		
1957	Holmgren	Stapediolysis		
1961	House	Introduction of the cochlear implant		
1963	Marquet	Stapedotomy		
1964	Shambaugh & Scott		Fluoride treatment	
1977	Tjelström	BAHA		
1980	Perkins	Laser stapedotomy		
1985	Stutzman & Petrovic		Biphosphonate treatment	

About the author

About the author

Rinze Anthony Tange MD, PhD
Associate Professor
Medical specialist in otolaryngology and otology at Utrecht University.

Rinze Tange was born in Utrecht, The Netherlands, on January 8, 1950. After secondary school (HBS-B), he studied medicine at the Utrecht University where he graduated in 1976. He then started his medical education in the specialty of otolaryngology by completing a four-year residency at the Erasmus University in Rotterdam. In 1977 Tange went to the Kresge Hearing Research Institute in Ann Arbor, Michigan, USA to study the inner ear anatomy research methods. He set up an otology laboratory for inner ear research in Rotterdam which was supported by Prof. E.H. Huizing and the Heinsius Houbold foundation. In 1983 he finished his thesis entitled Degenerative ototoxic changes in the cochlea as seen in microdissections and surface preparations. Tange was one of the first to demonstrate experimentally the toxic effects (ototoxicty) of the anticancer drug cisplatin on the hair-cells in the inner ear resulting in deafness. The thesis on this subject was defended in the University of Utrecht and was awarded with two awards: the Professor de Kleyn award 1987 (Best thesis 1980-1986) and the Duphar ENT-year award 1987.

In 1981, Tange moved from Rotterdam to the ENT department of the University of Amsterdam (head: Prof. L.B.W. Jongkees). Dr. Tange became interested in the treatment of hearing loss and went to Antwerpen to Prof. Jean Marquet to study his surgical approach of stapedectomy to treat otosclerosis. Since then Tange has performed nearly 1400 stapedectomies, with recovery of hearing in more than 94% of the cases. Over thirty publications on otosclerosis and stapedectomy appeared in the literature by Tange and his co-workers. In 1986, Tange performed the first implantation of the bone-conducting hearing aid called Audiant in The Netherlands. This type of implant was replaced by the Bone Anchored Hearing Aid (BAHA) later on. Over 300 BAHA implantations for conductive hearing loss were performed since then. In 2001, Tange founded the cochlear implant team at the Academic Medical Center in Amsterdam. He introduced an innovative non-invasive surgical approach to implant the cochlea prosthesis in profoundly deaf or severely hard of hearing patients. Over 300 CI implantations have been performed up until now. In 2003, Tange organized as president the 24th Politzer Society Meeting in the RAI iternational Congress Centre in Amsterdam ('Adam comes to A'dam'). In 2009, Tange was invited to join the ENT department of Utrecht University.

In 2010 he organized in the National Railway Museum in Utrecht the anniversity of '25 years Cochlear Implantations in Utrecht'.

Tange has published over 170 papers of which more than 100 are cited in PubMed and EMBASE free database search engines for text articles on life sciences and biomedical topics. He is the co-founder of the Dutch Journal of Otolaryngology / Head and Neck surgery, first published June 28, 1994 and has been editor from 1994-1999. Tange is founder member of European Academy of Otology and Neuro–Otology (EAONO) founded on 1996. In 2003, he was the President of the 24th Politzer Society Meeting in Amsterdam and organized this international congress. Tange is co-founder member of The LION Project a Global Visioconference Network for Otolaryngology. This Foundation was created in 2006 as a non-profit organization to promote medical and surgical high-quality continuing education programs.

Rinze Tange lives in Bussum, The Netherlands, together with Drs. Christine Dufour, neuro-psychologist. They have a son, Vincent Rinze Anthony (1980), and a daughter, Claire Helena (1983).

References

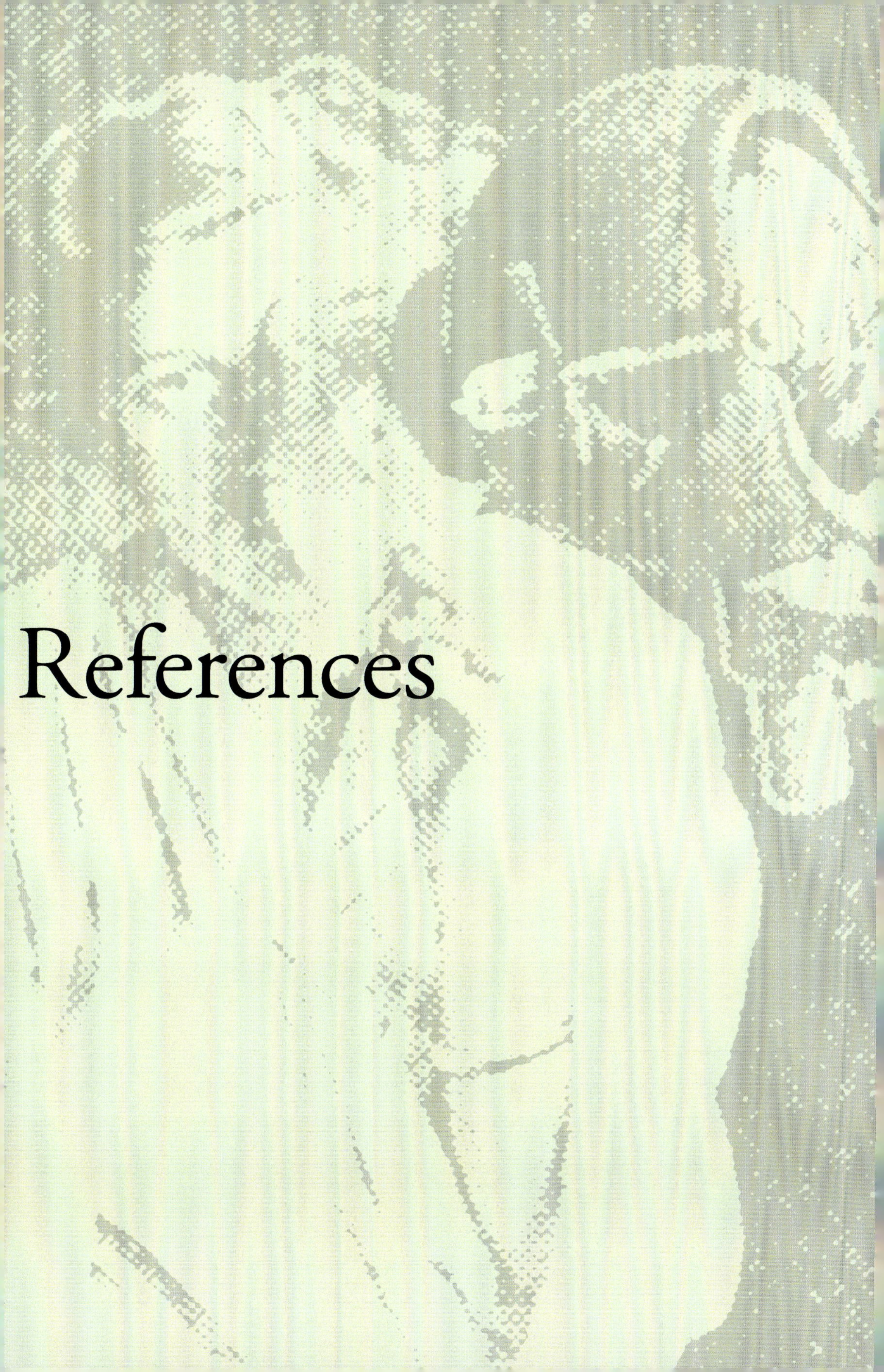

à Wengen DF. A new self-retaining titanium clip stapes prosthesis à Wengen: first clinical experience. Schweiz Med Wochenschr Suppl. 11, 2003

Abou Seree WR, Botrous RR, Mahmoud MA. Significance of high resolution CT scan in otosclerosis. Med J Cairo Univ 79(2):7-12, 2011

Alderston HA. Threphing of the stapedial footplate for otitis media sclerosa. Trans Am Otol Soc 7:60-63, 1898

Alonso JM, Chiarino A. Otosclerose ou otospongiose: influence exercee par la parathyroidectomie sur l'audition. Acta Oto-laryngol 27:123-135, 1939

Angeluscheff Z. Otosclerosis and ACTH. Acta Oto Laryngol 42:335-336, 1953

Angeluscheff Z, Coleman LL. Ultrasonics and otosclerosis; a new concept of its origin. AMA Arch Otolaryngol 58:398-404, 1953

Anonymus. Breguet's magneto-elektrischer Zündapparat. Engineering 193(7):17-20, 1869

Aubry M. La chirurgie de la surdité. Ann d'otolaryng 13:29, 1946

Bacon G, Blake CJ. A manual of otology. New York: Lea Brothers & Co, 1898

Ballance CA. Surgery of the temporal bone. Vol 2. London: MacMillan and Co, 1919

Balle V, Linthicum FH Jr. Histologically proven cochlear otosclerosis with pure sensorineural hearing loss. Ann Otol Rhinol Laryngol 93:105-111, 1984

Bárány TR. Die lndikationen zur Labyrinthoperation. Acta Laryngologica 6:260-288, 1924

Bárány TR. Worttabellen zur Horprufung. Verh Dtsch Otol Ges 19:110-113, 1910

Barton RT. The influence of pregnancy on otosclerosis. N Engl J Med 233:433-438, 1945

Barwell H. The service - X-ray treatment of otosclerosis 198:728, 1921

Bast F, Schrom T. First experiences with the new soft-clip piston as an alloplastic prosthesis during stapedotomy. Laryngorhinootologie 88:304-308, 2009

Bauer F. Stenosis of the auditory meatus following permeatal operations. J Laryngol Otol 70:475-484 , 1956

Beales PH: Otosclerosis. In: Kerr AG, Groves J (eds). Mean (SD) Scott-Brown's Otolaryngology, Vol 3, pp 44. London, England: Butterworths, 1987

Begall K, Zimmermann H. Rekonstruktion der gehorknochelchenkette mit Titan-implantaten. Laryngorhinootologie 79:139-145, 2000

Bergstrom G, Ivstam B. Vestibular disturbance after stapediolysis. Acta oto-laryng (Stockh.) 158: 328-334, 1960

Bernstein DS, Sadowsky N, Hagsted DM. Prevalence of osteoporosis in high and low fluoride areas of North Dakota. JAMA 198:499-505, 1966

Bernstien J, Gillis L. Otosclerosis treated with Sex hormones. Lancet 234:1368-1369, 1939

Bezold F. Ueberschau uber den gegenwärtigen stand der Ohrenheilkunde Wiesbaden: J.F. Bergmann, 1895

Bezold F. Otosklerosis. Lehrbuch der Ohrenheilkunde. Wiesbaden: J.F. Bergmann, 1906

Bezold F. Über die funktionelle Prüfung des menschlichen Gehörorgans. 3 volumes, Wiesbaden: J.F. Bergmann, 1897-1909

Blake CJ. Operation for the removal of the stapes. Boston Med & Surg J 127:469-470, 1892

Blohmke A. Otosklerose und Schwangerschaft. Arch f Ohren- ,Nasen- u Kehlkopfheilkunde 102:1-41, 1918

Bordes-Valls M. New approach for the treatment of otosclerosis. Arch Otolaryngol. 51:96-101, 1950

Bosatra A. Otosclerosis of the inner ear. A clinical study. J Laryngol Otol. 74: 209-216, 1960

Boucheron E. La mobilisation de l'etrier et son procede operatoire. Union Med Paris 46:412-413, 1888

Boucheron E. La mobilisation de l'etrier. Bull Med 2:1225, 1888

Boucheron E. Operation de la surdite otopiesique. C.R. Seances Acad Sci 106:1253-1256, 1888
Boumans LJ, Poublon RM. The detrimental effect of aminohydroxypropylidene bisphosphonate (APD) in otospongiosis. Eur Arch. Otorhinolaryngol 248:218-221, 1991
Boyce BF, Smith L, Fogelman I, Johnston E, Ralston S, Boyle IT. Focal osteomalacia due to low-dose diphosphonate therapy in Paget's disease. Lancet 1:821-824, 1984
Boyer EL, Kos CM. Vein plug stapedioplasty and bone conduction acuity. J Speech Hear Res 4:340-345, 1961
Brase C, Zenk J, Wurm J, Schick B, Iro H, Hornung J. Stapes surgery: first experiences with the new Soft-CliP piston. HNO 57:509-513, 2009
Bretlau P, Hansen HG, Causse JR, Causse JB. Otospongiosis: morphologic and microchemical investigation after NaF-treatment. Otolaryngol Head Neck Surg 89:646-650, 1981
Bretlau P, Causse JR, Causse JB, Hansen HJ, Johnsen NJ, Salomon G. Otospongiosis and sodium fluoride. A blind experimental and clinical evaluation of the effect of sodium fluoride treatment in patients with otospongiosis Ann. Otol Rhinol Laryngol 94:103-107, 1985
Bretlau P, Salomon G, Johnsen NJ. Otospongiosis and sodium fluoride. A clinical double-blind, placebo-controlled study on sodium fluoride treatment in otospongiosis. Am J Otol 10:20-22, 1989
Brickner SM. Infavourable influence of pregnancy and chronic progressive deafness. Cited by R. Frommel Jahresberichte über die fortschritte auf dem gebiete der geburtshilfe, Wiesbaden: J.F. Bergmann, 1911
Brondbo K, Hawke M, Abel SM, Alberti PW. The natural history of otosclerosis. A correlation of the volume and activity of the otosclerotic lesion with age. J Otolaryngol 12:163-168, 1983
Brookes GB. Vitamin D deficiency and otosclerosis. Otolaryngol Head Neck Surg 93:313-321, 1985

Brookler KH, Tanyeri H. Etidronate for the the neurotologic symptoms of otosclerosis: preliminary study. Ear Nose Throat J 76:371-376, 379-381, 1997

Brookler KH. Medical treatment of otosclerosis: rationale for use of bisphosphonates. Int Tinnitus J 14:92-96, 2008

Brooks D. Fenestration: A twenty-five-year evaluation. J Laryngol Otol 99:225-230, 1985

Browning GG. Management options: Fluoride In Scott-Brown Otosclerosis. In: Gleeson M (ed.). Scott-Brown's otorhinolaryngology: head and neck surgery, 7th edition, pp. 3453-3485. London: Hodder Arnold, 2008

Brühl G. Politzer A. Grundriss und Atlas der Ohrenheilkunde, Band XXIV, pp. 154-156. Munchen: J.F. Lehman's Verlag, 1905

Brunner H. Uber die Heilung von Bogengangsfisteln. Acta Otolaryngol 35:352, 1948

Burger H. Kunstmatige onderbreking der zwangerschap wegens otosklerose. Mededeling in de Ned Keel-Neus-Oorheelkundigen Vereniging 25 November 1923 Ned Tijdschr Geneeskd. 1924;68:252-255

Burger H. Interruption artificielle de grossesse a cause d'oto-sclerose. Acta Otolaryngol 7:133-138, 1925

Burrell SP, Cooper HC, Proops DW. The bone anchored hearing aid - The third option in otosclerosis. J Laryngol Otol 21:31-37, 1996

Calmels MN, Viana C, Wanna G, Marx M, James C, Deguine O, Fraysse B. Very far-advanced otosclerosis: stapedotomy or cochlear implantation. Acta Otolaryngol 127:574-578, 2007

Cathcart GC. The treatment of chronic deafness by the electrophonoide method of Zünd-Burguet. London: Milford, 1926

Cathcart GC. Discussion on otosclerosis. Societies' Proceedings British Medical Association 43(1): 68, 1927

Cathcart GC. The Treatment of Chronic Deafness by the Electrophonoïde Method of Zünd-Burguet. J Am Med Assoc 96(26):22-31, 1931

Cathcart GC. Seven Patients illustrating Alleviation of Deafness and Tinnitus by the Zund-Burguet Electrophonoide Method. Proc R Soc Med. May; 27(7): 897–899, 1934
Causse J. Stapedectomy and teflon-piston, teflon-interposition, repeated fenestrations. Ann Otolaryngol Chir Cervicofac 81:19-44, 1964
Causse JR, Shambaugh GE, Causse B, Bretlau P. Enzymology of otospongiosis and NaF therapy. Am J Otol 1:206-214, 1980
Causse JR, Uriel J, Berges J, Shambaugh GE Jr, Bretlau P, Causse JB. The enzymatic mechanism of the otospongiotic disease and NaF action on the enzymatic balance. Am J Otol 3:297-314, 1982
Causse JR, Causse JB, Uriel J, Berges J, Shambaugh GE Jr, Bretlau P. Sodium fluoride therapy. Am J Otol 14:482-490, 1993
Causse JB, Gherini S, Horn KL. Surgical treatment of stapes fixation by fiberoptic argon laser stapedotomy with reconstruction of the annular ligament. Otolaryngol Clin North Am 26:395-416, 1993
Causse JB, Vincent R, Michat M, Gherini S. Stapedius tendon reconstruction during stapedotomy: technique and results. Ear Nose Throat J 76:256-258, 260-269, 1997
Cawthorne T. Surgery for otosclerosis. Proc Royal Soc Med 63:491-499, 1950
Cawthorne T. The surgery of the temporal bone. Lecture at the Royal College of Surgeons of England, pp. 403-423, 1953
Cawthorne T. Stapes mobilization. J Laryngol Otol 72:281-283, 1958
Cawthorne T. Otosclerosis: The development of the surgical treatment of deafness. Proceedings of the Royal Society of Medicine 58:749-752, 1965
Cawthorne T. Julius Lempert a personal appreciation. Arch Otolaryngol 90:680-686, 1969
Chamyal PC, Ahluwalia KJS, Kessar RV. Sodium fluoride therapy in stapedial otosclerosis. Indian J Otolaryngol Head Neck Surg 42:150-153, 1990

Cho JJ, Yunker WK, Marck P, Marck PA. Effectiveness of the heat-activated nitinol smart piston stapes prosthesis in stapedectomy surgery. J Otolaryngol Head Neck Surg 40:8-13, 2011
Cody DT, Baker HL Jr. Otosclerosis: vestibular symptoms and sensorineural hearing loss. Ann Otol Rhinol Laryngol 87:778–796, 1978
Colletti V, Sittoni V, Fiorino FG. Stapedotomy with and without stapedius tendon preservation versus stapedectomy: long-term results. Am J Otol 9:136-141, 1988
Colletti V, Fiorino FG. Effect of sodium fluoride on early stages of otosclerosis. Am J Otol 12:195-198, 1991
Colletti V, Fiorino FG. Stapedotomy with stapedius tendon preservation: technique and long-term results. Otolaryngol Head Neck Surg 111:181-188, 1994
Crossland G, De R, Axon P. Far advanced otosclerosis and intractable benign paroxysmal positional vertigo treated with combined cochlear implantation and posterior semicircular canal occlusion. J Laryngol Otol Suppl 118:302-304, 2004
Cruise AS, Singh A, Quiney RE. Sodium fluoride in otosclerosis treatment: review. J Laryngol Otol 124:583-596, 2010
Cureoglu S, Baylan MY, Paparella MM. Cochlear otosclerosis. Curr Opin Otolaryngol Head Neck Surg 18:357-362, 2010
Daniel HJ. Stapedial otosclerosis and fluorine in drinking water. Arch Otolaryngol 90:585-589, 1969
Das TK, Susheela AK, Gupta IP, Dasarathy S, Tandon RK. Toxic effects of chronic fluoride ingestion on the upper gastrointestinal tract. Clin Gastroenterol 18:194-199, 1994
Davenport CB, Milles LB, Frink BL. The genetic factor in otosclerosis Arch Otolaryngol. 17(4): 503-548, 1933
Denker A. Otosklerose. Wiesbaden: J.F. Bergmann, 1904
DiBartolomeo JR, Ellis M. Argon laser in otology. Laryngoscope 90(11 Pt 1):1786-1796, 1980
Drury DW. Progressive deafness. The causative factors and specific diagnosis. Laryngoscope 34:545-550, 1926

Faraci G. Importanza acustica e funzionale delle mobilizzazione della staff; resultati di una nuova serie di operazioni. Arch Ital Otol Rinol Laryngol 9:209-221, 1899

Fish U. Tympanoplasty, mastoidectomy and stapes surgery, pp. 231-235. Stuttgart: Thieme, 1994

Floderus B. Bidrag till stigbygelankylosens operativa radikalbehandling. Nordiskt Medicinskt Arkiv 13:1-17, 1898

Fowler EP. Calcium, phosphorus and cholesterol in otosclerosis. Trans Am Otol Soc 13:77-83, 1930

Fowler EP. Calcium and phosphorus and phosphatase activity in otosclerosis. Arch Otolaryng 47:491, 1948

Fowler EP. Anterior crurotomy and mobilization of the ankylosed stapes footplate: introduction to a motion picture demonstration. 46:319-322, 1956

Freeman J. Progressive sensorineural hearing loss and cochlear otosclerosis: A prospective study. Laryngoscope 89:1487-1521, 1979

Freeman J. Otosclerosis and vestibular dysfunction. Laryngoscope 90:1481-1487, 1980

Frenckner P. Stapes mobilization: reflections and report of a new instrument. Acta Oto-laryngol 48:201-204, 1957

Frey H, Kriser A. Therapeutische Versuche mit Rontgenbehandlung bei Otosklerose. Verh d ges Deutsch Hals-, Nasen-, und Ohrenarzte. Kissingen, 1923

Frey H, Kriser A. Discussion in Klin. Wochenschrift 2 40:1862, 1923

Frey H, Kriser A. Therapeutische versuche mit Rontgenbehandlung bei Otosklerose. Zeitschrift für Hals-, Nasen- und Ohrenheilkunde 6:334-338, 1923

Frey H, Kriser A. Therapeutic Trials of the Rontgen Ray Treatment of Otosclerosis. Zeitschrift für Hals-, Nasen- und Ohrenheilkunde, 6(2): 334, 1924

Gantz BJ, Jenkins HA, Kishimoto S, Fisch U. Argon laser stapedotomy. Ann Otol Rhinol Laryngol 91:25-26, 1982

Gardner G, Robertson JH, Tomoda K, Clark WC. CO_2 laser stapedotomy: is it practical? Am J Otolaryngol 5:108-117, 1984

Garnett Passe ER. The fenestration operation for otosclerosis. Post graduate medical journal. 507-516, 1947

Gherini S, Horn KL, Causse JB, McArthur GR. Fiberoptic argon laser stapedotomy: is it safe? Am J Otol 14:283-289, 1993

Gill NW. The treatment of otosclerosis by mobilization of the stapes. J Laryngol Otol 72:807-818, 1958

Girgis IH. Preservation of the stapedius tendon in stapes surgery. J Laryngol Otol 880:733-742, 1966

Goodhill V. The use of cortisone in otosclerosis. Trans Am Acad Ophthalmol Otolaryngol 56:635-646, 1952

Goodhill V. Articulated polyethylene prosthesis with perichondral graft in stapedectomy. Rev Laryngol Otol Rhinol 82:305-320, 1961

Goodhill V. Stapedectomy - Its various forms. In: Stapes surgery for otosclerosis. V. Goodhill (ed), pp. 66-76. New York: Paul B. Hoeber, 1961

Gray AA. The Treatment of Otosclerotic and Similiar Types of Deafness by the Local Application of Thyroxine. Societies' Proceedings British Medical Association 45:741-759, 1935

Greifenstein A. Schwangerschaftsunterbrechung und unfruchtbarmachung aus gesundheitlichen Grunden bei Otosklerose. Zeitschrift fur hals nasen und ohrenheilkunde 46:344-362, 1939

Greifenstein A. Schwangerschaftsunterbrechung und unfruchtbarmachung aus gesundheitlichen Gründen bei Otosklerose. Hals-,Nasen-. u Ohrenartzt II 49:42, 1939

Gristwood RE. Obliterative otosclerosis. J Otolaryngol Soc Autr 2:40-48, 1966

Gristwood RE, Venables WN. Otosclerosis and pregnancy. Clin Otolaryngol Allied Sci 8:205-210, 1983

Guggenheim LK. On the diagnosis and treatment of otosclerosis. Am J Sur 42:156-169, 1938

Guild SR. Histologic otosclerosis. Ann Otol 53:246-252, 1944
Hammerschlag V. Zur Frage der Vererbbarkeit der Otosklerose. Monatsch f Ohren u Rhin 58:634-638, 1924
Havriliak D, Parisier SC. Cochlear otosclerosis presenting in children: a case report. Am J Otol 12:61-63, 1991
Hawkins JE Jr, Linthicum FH Jr, Johnsson LG. Cochlear and vestibular lesions in capsular otosclerosis as seen in microdissection. Ann Otol Rhinol Laryngol Suppl 87:1-40, 1978
Heimann B. Die Otosklerose. Monatsschrift fur ohrenheilkunde, 1909
Holleman IL, Harrill JA. Cochlear otosclerosis. Report of a case, with postmortem histologic findings. Laryngoscope 77:493-507, 1967
Holmgren G. Till otosclerosens kirurgiska behandlung. Nordiskt tidskrift Oto-Laryngol 2:217, 1917
Holmgren G. Some experiences in the surgery of otosclerosis. Acta Otolaryngol 5:460-466, 1923
Holmgren G. Present-day surgery of otosclerosis. Acta Otolaryngol 36:19-25, 1948
Holmgren L. Stapediolysis in otosclerosis. Acta Oto-laryngol 48:219-233, 1957
Holmgren L. Mobilization and stapediolysis. Acta Oto-laryngol 158:316-327, 1960
House HP, Sheehy JL. Stapes surgery: selection of the patient. Ann Otol Rhinol Laryngol 70:1062-1068, 1962
Hubby LM. Treatment of deafness with sonorous vibrations by the Zünd Burguet method. New York Med. Rec, 1914
Huber AM, Schrepfer T, Eiber A. Clinical evaluation of the NiTiBOND stapes prosthesis, an optimized shape memory alloy design. Otol Neurotol 33(2):132-6.2011
Hutchinson CA. Labyrinthine fenestration -The present position J Laryngol Otol 61:567-585, 1946
Hutchinson CA. Cortisone in fenestration surgery. Clinical note. J Laryngol Otol 68:189-190, 1954

Hyman SR. For the world to hear: a biography of Dr. Howard P. House, pp. 255-258. Pasadena: Hope Publishing House, 1990

Iurato S, Ettorre GC, Onofri M, Davidson C. Very far advanced otosclerosis. Am J Otol 13:482-487, 1992

Jack FL. Remarkable improvement of hearing by removal of the stapes. Trans Amer Otol 5:284-305, 1892

Jack FL. Further observations on removal of the stapes. Trans Amer Otol 5:474-487, 1893

Jack FL. Remarks on stapedectomy. Trans Amer Otol 6:102-106, 1894

Jaulin M. Traitement de l'otite par les Rayons X. Arch d'electr Med 231:92, 1908

Jeffcoate TN. Indications for therapeutic abortion. Brit Medical Journ 1:581-588, 1960

Jenkins GJ. Otosclerosis: Certain clinical features and experimental operative procedures. Transactions of the XVIIth international Congress of Medicine in London Section XVI part 1 Otology:609-918, 1913

Jenkins GJ, Edin CM, Eng FRCS. The treatment of otosclerosis. J Laryngol Otol 29:520-523, 1914

Jones MF. Critical survey of the Lempert endaural fenestration operation. Laryngoscope 57:263-71, 1947

Jongkees LBW. Fenestratie van het labyrinth. N.T.v G. 93.IV 42:3547-3553, 1949

Jongkees LBW. Preaural tympanic surgery (Popper's approach). Acta Otolaryngol 38:498-504, 1950

Juers AL. Stapedioplasty: A new concept for stapes surgery. Laryngoscope 69:1180-1193, 1959

Juers AL. Julius Lempert His Legacy to Otology. Arch Otolaryngol 90: 700-701, 1969

Keen JA. The treatment of the Ménière syndrome by the Zünd Burguet electrophonoïde vibromassage. The Lancet 6:285-286, 1932

Kennedy DW, Hoffer ME, Holliday M. The effects of etidronate disodium on progressive hearing loss from otosclerosis. Otolaryngol Head Neck Surg 109:461-467, 1993

Kerr GS, Hoffman GS. Fluoride therapy for otosclerosis. Ear Nose Throat J 68:426, 428-429, 1989

Kessel J. Ueber die durchschneidung des steigbugelmuskels beim menschene und uber die extraction des steigbugels, respectieve der columella bei thieren. Arch f Ohrenh 11:199-217, 1876

Kessel J. Die Erfolge der Extraction des Stapes. Arch f Ohrenh 12:237, 1877

Kessel J. Uber die vordere Tenotomie, Mobilisierung und Extraction des Steigbugels. Jena: Fisher Verlag, 1894

Klabenes FJ. Pregnancy complicating otosclerosis. Nebr State Med J 49:550-55, 1964

Knox GW, Reitan H. Shape-memory stapes prosthesis for otosclerosis surgery. Laryngoscope 115:1340-1346, 2005

Korner O. Lehrbuch der Ohren-,Nasen- und Kehlkopf - Krankheiten, pp. 338-343. Wiesbaden: J.F. Bergman, 1914

Krumpholz K. On the teflon-wire-piston technic. Monatsschr Ohrenheilkd Laryngorhinol 102:63-68, 1968

Kwok P, Fisch U, Strutz J, Jacob P. Comparative electron microscopic study of the surface structure of gold, Teflon, and titanium stapes prostheses. Otol Neurotol 22:608-613, 2001

Kwok P, Fisch U, Strutz J, May J. Stapes surgery: how precisely do different prostheses attach to the long process of the incus with different instruments and different surgeons? Otol Neurotol 23:289-295, 2002

Laughlin HH. Eugenical sterilization in the United States, pp. 1-502. Chicago: Psychopathic Laboratory of the Municipal Court of Chicago, 1922

Lavrand H. Phonatory Massage in Progressive Deafness. Arch Internat Laryngol, d'Otol et de Rhinol p.140, 1913

Leea TCR, Aviva RI, Chenb JM, Nedzelskib JM, Foxa AJ, Symonsa SP. CT Grading of Otosclerosis. AJNR 30:1435-1439, 2009

Leicher H. Innere sekretion und krankheiten des ohres Leipzig: Kabitzsch, 1928

Lempert J. Improvement of hearing in cases of otosclerosis. A new one-stage surgical technique. Arch Otolaryn 28:42-97, 1938

Lempert J. Endaural fenestration of the external semicircular canal for restoration of hearing in cases of otosclerosis. Arch Otolaryn 31:711-779, 1940

Lempert J. Lempert fenestra Nov-Ovalis with mobile stopple. Arch Otolaryn 41: l, 1945

Lempert J. Transtympanosympathectomy: a surgical technic for the relief of tinnitus aurium. Arch Otol 43:199-212 , 1946

Lempert J. The Permanently Patent Fenestra Nov-Ovalis. Laryngoscope 61:215, 1951

Lesinski SG, Stein JA. CO2 laser stapedotomy. Laryngoscope 99:20-24, 1989

Lindsay JR. Healing of Experimental Labyrinthine Fistulas: Further Observation. Arch Otolaryngol 46:584-600, 1947

Linthicum FH, Filipo R, Brody S. Sensorineural hearing loss due to cochlear otospongiosis: theoretical considerations of etiology. Otolaryngol Clin North Am 84:125-134, 1978

Lippy WH, Berenholz LP, Schuring AG, Burkey JM. Does pregnancy affect otosclerosis? Laryngoscope 115:1833-1836, 2005

Lumsden RB. The fenestration operation: A review based on an analysis of 139 operations. J Laryngol Otol 72:102-117, 1958

Manasse P. Die ostitis chronica metaplastica der menschlichen labyrinthkapsel (otosklerose, stapesankylose, spongiosierung der labyrinthkapsel). Wiesbaden: J.F. Bergmann, 1912

Manasse P. Neue untersuchingen zur otosklerosenfrage. Zschr Ohrenheilk 82:234-243, 1922

Marquet J. Le syndrome de suridite du a une deficience de la prothese stapedienne. Congres Soc Franc d'ORL, pp 151-160. Paris : Libraire Arnett, Comptes Rendues des Seances, 1965

Marquet J. Technique of stapedotomy. In: Otosclerosis Proceedings of International Workshop on Otosclerosis. R Fillipo (ed.), pp. 83-87. Amsterdam/Milan: Kugler Publications and Ghedini Editoria, 1990

Maurice A. Traitement de la Surdité par la Ré-éducation de l'Ouïe, 1912

Maurer H. Biochemical aspects of otosclerosis. Arch Otolaryngol 85:24-28, 1967

McGee TM. Lasers in otology. Otolaryngol Clin North Am 22:233-238, 1989

McKenzie W, Rainer EH. The Rosen operation; early experience. J Laryngol Otol. 71:655-666, 1957

Merkus P,van Loon MC, Smit CF, Smits C, de Cock AFC, Hensen EF. Decision making in advanced otosclerosis: An evidence-based strategy. Laryngoscope 121:1935-1941, 2011

Meurman Y, Meurman O. Stapes mobilization in otosclerosis; primary results and a review of sixty-three cases. AMA Arch Otolaryngol 62:164-172, 1955

Meurman Y. Surgery in Otosclerosis. Acta Otolaryngol 49:45-65, 1958

Miles Foxen EH. Relief of deafness by stapes mobilization. Brit Med J 2(5112):1588-1561, 1958

Miot C. De la mobilisation de l'etrier. Rev Laryngol d'Otol Rhinol 10:113-130, 1890

Mirvish L. Otosclerosis; a metabolic disorder. J Laryngol Otol 45:449-464, 1930

Morawiec-Baijda A, Durko T. Vertigo and objective vestibular symptoms in computer analysis of ENG in otosclerotic patients and after stapes operations. Otolaryngol Pol 54:415-421, 2000

Morrison AW. Treatment of otosclerosis by stapedectomy. Br Med J 130:1804-1807, 1962

Moure EJ. De la mobilisation de l'etrier. Rev Laryngol d'Otol Rhinol 10:225-232, 1890

Mudry A, Tjellström A. Historical background of bone conduction hearing devices and bone conduction hearing aids. In: Implantable bone conduction hearing aids. Kompis M, Caversaccio MD (eds.) , vol 71, pp. 1-9. Adv Otorhinolaryngol. Basel: Karger, 2011

Nager FR, Fraser JS. On bone formation in the scala tympani of otosclerotics. J Laryngol Otol 53(3):173-180, 1938

Nassuphis VP. Ergebnisse der otosklerose-operation. Duraluftung uber dem Tegmen Tympani nach Wittmaack. Acta Oto-laryngologica 39: 217–221, 1951

Ortloff H. Uber therapeutische versuche mit Rontgenstrahlen bei der otosklerose. Eur Arch Otolaryngol 9:233-244, 1913

Palva T. Argon laser in otosclerosis surgery. Acta Otolaryngol 104:153-157, 1987

Parahy CH, Linthicum FH. Relationship of spiral ligament hyalinization to sensorineural hearing loss. Laryngoscope 93:717-720, 1983

Parnes LS, McClure JA. Posterior semicircular canal occlusion in the normal hearing ear. Otolaryngol Head Neck Surg 104:52-57, 1991

Passow K. Operative anlegung einer offnung in die mediale paukenhohlewand by stapes ankylosis. Verh Dtsch Otol Ges 6:43-144, 1897

Pearson E. The effect of pregnancy on otosclerosis. Ann West Med Surg 5:477-482, 1951

Perkins RC. Laser stapedotomy for otosclerosis. Laryngoscope 90:228-240, 1980

Petrovic A, Shambaugh GE Jr. Promotion of bone calcification by sodium fluoride: short-term experiments on new-born rats using tetracyclyne labeling. Arch Otolaryngol 83:104-112, 1966

Podoshin L, Gertner R, Fradis M. Oral contraceptive pills and clinical otosclerosis. Int J Gynaecol Obstet 15:554-555, 1978

Politzer A. Ueber Anchylose des steigbügels mit dem ovalen fenster. AllgWien Med Ztg 7:220-221, 1862

Politzer A. Lehrbuch der Ohrenheilkunde. Stuttgart: Enke, 1878
Politzer A. The extraction of the stapes. J Laryngol Otol 15:66-68, 1900
Popper O. Fenestration of the labyrinth Part I & Part II. J Laryngol Otol 61:24-37, 441-458, 1946
Poulsen IPV. Popper's operation for otosclerosis. Acta Otolaryngol 43:466-473, 1953
Precechtel A. Determination of the effect of pregnancy on the activation of otosclerosis. Acta Otolaryngol 63:121-127, 1967
Pusalkar AG, Steinbach E. Gold implants in middle ear reconstructive surgery. In: Yanagihara N,Suzuki J (eds.) Transplants and implants in Otology II, pp. 111-113. Amsterdam/New York: Kugler Publications, 1992
Rama-López J, Cervera-Paz FJ, Manrique M. Cochlear Implantation of Patients with Far-Advanced Otosclerosis. J Otol Neurotol 27:153-158, 2006
Rambo JHT. Factors affecting healing following temporal bone surgery. Laryngoscope 6:810-845, 1956
Raoult A. Reducation (anakinisie) de l'oule, par la methode Electro-Phonoide. Gaz Hop 85:904-906, 1912
Raoult A. Auditory re-education: remote results of auditory re-education. Arch Internat Laryngol, d'Otol et de Rhinol 138, 1913
Raut VV, Toner JG, Kerr AG. Stevenson M. Management of otosclerosis in de UK. Clin Otolaryngol 27:113-119, 2002
Redfors YD, Möller C. Otosclerosis: Thirty-year follow-up after surgery. Ann. Otol. Rhinol. Laryngol. 120:608-614, 2011
Riechelmann H, Tholen M, Keck T, Rettinger G. Perioperative glucocorticoid treatment does not influence early post-laser stapedotomy hearing thresholds. Am J Otol 21:809-812, 2000
Riggs BL, Hodgson SF, Hoffman DL, Kelly PJ, Johnson KA, Taves D. Treatment of primary osteoporosis with fluoride and calcium. Clinical tolerance and fracture occurrence. JAMA 243:446-449, 1980

Riskaer N. Response of otosclerosis and adhesive otitis to treatment with corticotrophin. AMA Arch Otolaryngol 55(3):343-349, 1952
Riscardson J. X-ray as an advance in the treatment of impaired hearing. Eye Ear Nose Throat Mon 2:578, 1923
Rollin H. Bericht uber die ersten zwanzig operierten Otosklerosefalle. European Archives of Oto-Rhino-Laryngology 138(1): 6-19, 1933
Rollin H. Die Otosklerose und ihre operative behandlung. European Archives of Oto-Rhino-Laryngology 156(2-6): 248-252, 1950
Rosen S. Is it Possible to Cover the Fenestra Nov-Ovalis with Shrapnell's Membrane ? Arch Otolaryngol 49:529-534, 1949
Rosen S. Palpation of stapes for fixation: preliminary procedure to determine fenestration suitability in otosclerosis. AMA Arch Otolaryngol 56:610-615, 1952
Rosen S. Mobilization of the stapes to restore hearing in otosclerosis. New York State J Med 53:2650-2653, 1953
Rotteveel LJC, Proops DW, Ramsden RT, Saeed SR, van Olphen AF, Mylanus EAM. Cochlear implantation in 53 patients with otosclerosis: demographics, computed tomographic scanning, surgery, and complications. Otol Neurotol 25:943-952, 2004
Rüedi L, Schneider R, Egli P, Perk P. Results of the retro-aural two stages fenestration operation for hearing impairment due to otosclerosis. Acta Oto laryngologica 40(3-4):226-238, 1951-1952
Rüedi L. Fortschritte in der chirurgischen Behandlung der otosklerotischen Schwerhörigkeit; Stapesmobillsation, Fenestration der Stapesfussplatte oder transmeatale Fenestration des horizontalen Bogenganges mit Incudopexie? Schweiz Med Wochenschr 89:8-13, 1954
Rüedi L. Neuentwicklung der Chirurgie der Otosklerose. Dtsch med Wochenschr 86:2305-2309, 1961
Rüedi L. Histopathologic confirmation of labyrinthine otosclerosis. Arch Otolaryngol 83:160, 1966

Sabitha R, Ramalingam R, Ramalingam KK, Sivakumaran TA, Ramesh A. Genetics of otosclerosis. J Laryngol Otol 111:109-112, 1997

Sachdev KB, Bhatia ML. Observations with a new conservative treatment in otosclerosis. Indian J Otolaryngol Head Neck Surg 16:174-190, 1962

Salem W. O uso do molde acrilico perfurado em fenestração. RBORL 19(1): 1-3, 1951

Salvinelli F, Trivelli M, Greco F, Linthicum FH jr. Otosclerosis and cochlear otosclerosis: A post mortem study on temporal bones. Eur Rev Med Pharmacol Sci 179:179-182, 1999

Sando I, Hemenway WG, Hildyard V, English GM. Cochlear otosclerosis: a human temporal bone report. Ann Otol Rhinol Laryngol 77:23-36, 1968

Saper RB, Phillips RS, Sehgal A, Khouri N, Davis RB, Paquin J, Thuppil V, Kales SN. Lead, mercury, and arsenic in US- and Indian-manufactured ayurvedic medicines sold via the Internet. J Am Med Assoc 300:915-923, 2008

Scheer AA. Observations of five hundred cases of transtympanic mobilization of the stapes. AMA Arch Otol 65:245-254, 1957

Schmalix J. Praktische bedeutung des Ultra-schalles für de Oto-Rhinologie. Med Klein 45:564, 1950

Schuknecht HF. Oleksiuk S. The metal prosthesis for stapes ankylosis. AMA Arch Otolaryngol 71:287-295, 1960

Schuknecht HF. Cochlear otosclerosis. Eur Arch Otorhinolaryngol 222:79-84, 1979

Schwartz G. Die Rontgenstrahlen im dienste der Ohrenheilkunde. Med f Ohrh 44:675, 1910

Schwartze H. Pathology der synostose des steigbügels. Arch. Für Orhrenheilk. Vol. 5 1 : 257-271. 1870

Schwartze H. Handbuch der Ohrenheilkunde. Leipzig: verlag von F.C.W. Vogel, 1893.

Sellari-Franceschini S, Ravecca F, De Vito A Berrettini S. Progressive sensorineural hearing loss in cochlear otosclerosis. Acta Otorhinolaryngol Ital 18:59-65, 1998

Sexton S. Operation for deafness and tinnitus, due to immobilization of the ossicles and for otorrhea. Br Med J 11:69-70, 1890
Shambaugh GE Jr. The diagnosis and treatment of active cochlear otosclerosis. J Laryngol Otol 301-314, 1971
Shambaugh GE Jr. Fenestration operation for otosclerosis. JAMA 130:999-1006, 1946
Shambaugh GE Jr. Fenestration operation for otosclerosis: Experimental investigation and clinical observations in 2,100 operations over a period of 10 years. Acta Otolaryngol 79:1-101, 1949
Shambaugh GE jr. Long term results fenestration surgery. Acta Otolaryngol 40:180-191, 1951
Shambaugh GE Jr, Scott A. Sodium fluoride for arrest of otosclerosis. Arch Otolaryngol 80:263-270, 1964
Shambaugh GE Jr, Glasscock ME III. In: Surgery of the ear, pp. 455-516. Philadelphia: W.B. Saunders, 1980
Shambaugh GE Jr. Julius Lempert and the fenestration operation. Am J Otol 15:247-452, 1995
Shea JJ, Sanabria F, Smith GDL. Teflon piston operation for otosclerosis. Arch Otolaryngol 76 :516-521, 1962
Shea JJ Jr. The teflon piston operation for otosclerosis. Laryngoscope 73:508-509, 1963
Shea JJ. Forty years of stapes surgery. Am J Otol 19:52-55, 1998
Siebenmann F. Traitement chirugical de la sclerose otique. Cong Int Med sec Otol 13:170, 1900
Siebenmann F. Totaler knöchener verschluss beider labyrinth fenster und labyrithitis serosa infolge progresiver spongiosierung Verh Dtsch Otol Ges 20:267-274, 1911
Siirala U. Contribution to the technique of fenestration. Acta Oto-Laryngol 42(3):275-279, 1952
Silverstein H. Laser stapedotomy minus prosthesis (laser STAMP): a minimally invasive procedure. Am J Otol 19:277-282, 1998

Silverstein H, Hester TO, Rosenberg SI, Deems DA. Preservation of the stapedius tendon in laser stapes surgery. Laryngoscope. 108:1453-1458, 1998

Silverstein H, Jackson LE, Conlon WS, Rosenberg SI, Thompson JH Jr. Laser Stapedotomy Minus Prosthesis (Laser STAMP): Absence of Refixation. Otol Neurotol 23:152-157, 2002

Silverstein H, Hoffmann KK, Thompson JH Jr, Rosenberg SI, Sleeper JP. Hearing outcome of laser stapedotomy minus prosthesis (STAMP) versus conventional laser stapedotomy. Otol Neurotol 25:106-111, 2004

Simson Hall I. Fenestration operation for otosclerosis. Br Med J 2:647-649, 1946

Skoog T. Surgery for otosclerosis. Nord Med 49:353, 1953

Schmidt E. Heredity and Pregnancy in Otosclerosis. Arch. Ohr-, u.s.w., Heilk., 136, 188-201. 1933

Smyth GDL, Hassard TH. Hearing aids poststapedectomy: incidence and timing. Laryngoscope 96:356-358, 1986

Sohier Bryant W, JS Fraser. The etiology of otosclerosis. Laryngol Rhino Otol 30(10):389-397, 1915

Sourdille M. On the surgical treatment of Otosclerosis. J Laryngol Otol 23:601-614, 1930

Sourdille M. Nouvelles techniques operatoires pour le traitement des surdites chroniques progressives ou otosclerose Acta Otolaryngol 15:13-34, 1931

Sourdille M. New technique in the surgical treatment of severe and progressive deafness from otosclerosis. Bulletin of The New York Academy of Medicine 13:673-691, 1937

Sourdille M. Tendances évolutives de la fenestration. Paris: Masson & Cie, 1955

Steger F, Schmer B, Strube W, Becker T. Forced sterilisation based on the law for the prevention of hereditarily diseased offspring: The role of the Heil- und Pflegeanstalt (State Hospital) Günzburg: Nervenarzt, 2011

Stein C. Konstitutionspathologie in der Ohrenheilkunde Zentr. F Hals, Nasen u Ohrenh 6:224, 1924

Stein C. The influence of sexual development and disorders on the etiology of otosclerosis. In : Wien Klin Wochenschr, Abstraced by F. C. ORMEROD. Journal Otol & Larryngol 40(10) : 678, 1925

Stevenson WC, Wilson TG. The rationale of the radium treatment of middle ear deafness, with a preliminary report of its effect on chronic hyperplastic otitis media. Ir J Med Sc 1:630-634, 1926

Stutzmann JJ, Petrovic AG. Diphosphonates for otospongiosis. Am J Otol 6:89-95, 1985

Sultan A. A histoire de l'otolgie. In: M Barbaix, J Willemot Naissance et developpement de l'Oto-rhino-laryngologie dans l'histoire de la medicine, pp. 1344-1364. Acta ORL Belg, 1981

Swartz JD, Mandell DW, Berman SE, Wolfson RJ, Marlowe FI, Popky GL. Cochlear otosclerosis (otospongiosis): CT analysis with audiometric correlation. Radiology 155:147-150, 1985

Tange RA, de Bruijn AJ, Grolman W. Experience with a new pure gold piston in stapedotomy for cases of otosclerosis. Auris Nasus Larynx 25:249-253, 1998

Tange RA, Schimanski G, van Lange JW, Grolman W, Zuur LC. Reparative granuloma seen in cases of gold piston implantation after stapes surgery for otosclerosis. Auris Nasus Larynx 29:7-10, 2002

Tange RA, Grolman W. Late postoperative hearing results after stapedotomy. Int Adv Otol 5: 323-326, 2009

Tange RA, Grolman W, Dreschler WA. What to do with the other ear after cochlear implantation. Cochlear Implants Int. 10(1):19-24, 2009

Tjellström A, Lindström J, Hallén O, Albrektsson T, Brånemark PI. Osseointegrated titanium implants in the temporal bone. A clinical study on bone-anchored hearing aids. Am J Otol 2:304-310, 1981

Tos M. Surgical solutions for conductive hearing loss, pp 86-109. Stuttgart/New York: Thieme, 2000

Toynbee J. Diseases of the ear. London: Churchill, 1860

Toynbee J. Anchylosis of the stapes to the fenestra ovalis. pp : 289-309 in : The Disease of the Ear: Nature, Diagnoses and Treatment. Philadelphia: Blanchard and Lea, 1860

Tweedie AR. Otosclerosis: Some points in its etiology, diagnose, and treatment. Lancet 19:1808-1810, 1908

Uppal S, Bajaj Y, Coatesworth AP. Otosclerosis 2: the medical management of otosclerosis. Int J Clin Pract 64:256-265, 2010

Valiathan MS. Ayurveda: Putting the House in Order. Current Science Indian Academy of Sciences 90:5-6, 2006

Valiathan MS. Bioethics and ayurveda. Indian J Med Ethics 5:29-30, 2008

Valvassori GE. Laminography of the ear in otosclerosis. Rev Laryngol Otol Rhinol (Bord) 84:770-778, 1963

Valvassori GE. Radiologic diagnosis of cochlear otosclerosis. Laryngoscope 75:1563-1571, 1965

Valvassori GE. Imaging of the temporal bone. In: Glasscock ME, Shambaugh GE Jr (eds.) Surgery of the ear, 4th edition, pp. 110-111. Philadelphia: W.B. Saunders, 1990

Vartiainen E, Karjalainen S, Nuutinen J, Suntioninen S, Pellinen P. Effect of drinking water fluoridation on hearing of patients with otosclerosis in a low fluoride area: a follow-up study. Am J Otol 15:545-548, 1994

Vartiainen E, Vartiainen J. The influence of drinking water on the long-term hearing results of stapedectomy. Clin Otolaryngol and allied Sciences 22:34-36, 1997

Vasalva A. De aure humane tractus. Bononiae: Pisarii, 1724

Venters RS. Stapes mobilization. J Laryngol Otol 72:284-291, 1958

Voss O. Diskussion nach Vortrag von F. Siebenmann: "Uber die Anfangsstad und fieber der Natur progressive Spongiosierung der Labyrinthkapsel ". Verh Deutsch Otol Ges 21:193, 1912

Voss O. Ultraschallwellen im Dienste der Behandlung chronischer Schwerhörigkeit, Arch f Ohren-,Nasen- u Kehlkopfheilkunde

Walsh TE. The effect of pregnancy on the deafness due to otosclerosis. Am Med Assoc 154:1407-1409, 1945

Warwick HL, Stevenson HM. Is there an endocrine factor in otosclerosis? Acta otolaryng 9:317-324, 1926

Warwick HL, Stevenson HM. X-ray therapy in otosclerosis. Acta Otolaryng 9 : 339-343, 1926

Wazen JJ, Young DL, Farrugia MC, Chandrasekhar SS, Ghossaini SN, Borik J, Soneru C, Spitzer JB. Successes and complications of the Baha system. Otol Neurotol 29:1115-1119, 2008

Waugh Smith H. Effect of pregnancy on otosclerosis. Arch Otolaryngol. 48(2): 159-170, 1948

Webster JHD. X-ray treatment of otosclerosis. The Lancet 24:647-649, 1921

Weersma P. Fenestratie bij otosclerose. N.T.v.G. 91.II. 15:856-863, 1947

Weichbold V, Zorowka P. Zangssterilisation bie erblicher taubheit im dritten reich. HNO 17:1-18, 2008

Wittmaack K. Uber die pathologisch-anatomischen und pathologischphysiologischen Grundlagen der nichteitrigen Erkrankungsprozesse des inneren Ohres und des Hörnerven Arch f Ohren-,Nasen- u Kehlkopfheilkunde, pp. 71-136, 1916

Wittmaack K. Die otosklerose auf grund eigener forschungen. Jena, Gustaf Fischer, 1919

Wittmaack K. The pathogenesis of otosclerosis. Arch Otolaryngol 14:186-194, 1931

Wittmaack K. Betrachtungen zum Otoskleroseproblem. Acta Otolaryngol 18:217-264, 1933

Wittmaack K. Uber die operative behandlung der Otosklerose mit duraluftung an tegmen tympani. Klin Wschr 12:658-662, 1933

Wolf D. Über den einfluss der schwangerschaft auf der gehörorgan. In : Uber den gegenwartigen stand der otosclerose. Blaus Enzyklopaedie S 360, Wiesbaden: J.F. Bergmann, 1895

Yaşil S, Cömlekçi A, Güneri A. Further hearing loss during osteoporosis treatment with etidronate. Postgrad Med J 74:363-436, 1998

Yearsley M. The Zünd Burguet treatment. To the editor of the lancet. The Lancet 28:740, 1936

Yearsley M. Comment on Otosclerosis Treated with Sex Hormones . J Laryngol Otol Vol. 54 : 132, 1939

Yongkang Ou, Zhigang Zhang, Suijun Chen, Yaodong Xu, Haidi Yang, Yan Ma, Yiqing Zheng. Cochlear otosclerosis: 3 cases report and literature review. Journal of clinical otorhinolaryngology, head, and neck surgery 23:14-16, 2009

Zollner H. Discussion: Arch f Ohren-, Nasen- u Kehlkopfheilkunde 165:2-6, 1954

Zollner F. Experiences with the Rosen technic of stapes mobilization. Z Laryngol Rhinol Otol 38:410-421, 1959

Zünd-Burguet A. Principes d'Anaconsie (rééducation auditive). Paris: Maloine, 1913

Zuur CL, de Bruijn AJ, Lindeboom R, Tange RA. Retrospective analysis of early postoperative hearing results obtained after stapedotomy with implantation of a new titanium stapes prosthesis. Otol Neurotol 24:863-867, 2003